The Reluctant
Caregivers

The Reluctant Caregivers

Learning to Care for a Loved One
with Alzheimer's

Anne Hendershott

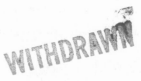

BERGIN & GARVEY
Westport, Connecticut • London

Library of Congress Cataloging-in-Publication Data

Hendershott, Anne B.
    The reluctant caregivers : learning to care for a loved one with Alzheimer's
    / Anne Hendershott.
      p. cm.
    Includes bibliographical references and index.
    ISBN 0–89789–711–0 (alk. paper)
    1. Alzheimer's disease—Patients—Care. 2. Alzheimer's disease—Popular
works. I. Title.

    RC523.2.H456 2000
    362.1'96831—dc21   99–046149

British Library Cataloguing in Publication Data is available.

Library of Congress Catalog Card Number: 99–046149
ISBN: 0–89789–711–0

First published in 2000

Bergin & Garvey, 88 Post Road West, Westport, CT 06881
An imprint of Greenwood Publishing Group, Inc.
www.greenwood.com

Printed in the United States of America

The paper used in this book complies with the
Permanent Paper Standard issued by the National
Information Standards Organization (Z39.48–1984).

10 9 8 7 6 5 4 3 2

Contents

Acknowledgments

I owe a special debt of gratitude to Marge Galante, RN, director of the Glenner Alzheimer's Family Day Care Center in San Diego, California. Marge provided encouragement and support throughout our family caregiving journey. Her kindness to Katharine and her willingness to "share the caring" with us will always be treasured.

I am also grateful to Monsignor Dan Dillabough, who reminded us often of the special grace that God gives to caregivers. His prayers and support sustained us throughout our caregiving years.

This book evolved from the generosity of many. Anne Hawkin and Jan Fain provided insightful suggestions and helpful criticisms at the early stage of this project. At Bergin and Garvey, I was fortunate to work with Lynn Taylor, who recognized the need for this book, and with Heidi Straight, whose superb editing ability greatly enhanced the writing.

A very special thank you to my husband Dana, and our God-given children, Heidi and Jonathan. I am especially grateful to Jonathan for his willingness to share his experiences to help others understand the sacrifices that caregiving children must make.

And, finally, to Katharine, who taught us that even reluctant caregivers can learn to care. We cherish the final gift of her presence in our lives.

Introduction: Becoming a Caregiver

It is often difficult, looking back on the life of one who develops Alzheimer's disease, to be able to say, "yes, it started then." Even today, my husband, Dana, and I often sit and look through our photo albums for signs of when his mother began to slip away. We look closely at pictures of Katharine that were taken during past holiday visits or at our children's graduations and birthday parties. We are always looking for clues of her impending disease to try and determine exactly when it began.

With the luxury of hindsight, we can now recall some signs in her behavior that we probably should have seen. Still, we cannot find a single picture which might have hinted at Katharine's early Alzheimer's disease. We look closely at her face in pictures taken from one Christmas to the next. Sometimes, when we look especially carefully at her eyes, we think we can see the beginnings of the dimming that progressed ever so slowly.

In many ways, the creation of the caregiving role may be viewed as a similar kind of progression, because caregiving often has an indefinite beginning. Many of those who have become caregivers to elderly parents or spouses are not quite sure exactly when they assumed the role. As a child or a spouse of an impaired loved one, the caregiver may be surprised to look back and be unable to remember exactly when the caregiving began. For the child of an impaired parent, the role change was so subtle that the caregiving child has no idea when the parent became the child and the child became the parent. Likewise, for many spouses of Alzheimer's victims, caregiving has an almost imperceptible onset because providing assistance with transportation, banking, and household chores are often assumed by spouses as part of their marital role. Because of this, spouses of impaired individuals tend not to recognize their early days of caregiving as unique from their role as spouse, until they begin providing personal care. As a result, it is often impossible for caregivers to say, "yes, this was when I became the caregiver." Most often, when a parent or spouse has Alzheimer's disease, the caregiving child or spouse evolves into the role in subtle ways.

Caregivers may begin their caretaking roles by providing incidental help on an occasional basis. Perhaps in the early days, even before caregivers have acknowledged that there might be something wrong with the parent or spouse, they may offer some help with simple tasks like grocery shopping or gardening. Later, caregivers might progress to the point where they are providing additional services because they realize that the parent or spouse needs help with household tasks. And, quite unexpectedly, and sometimes reluctantly, the person giving help has evolved to the point where he or she has become the caregiver. At this point, caregiving activities may have gradually expanded to the point where they have, in effect, restructured and largely taken over the caregivers' lives, displacing or reducing previous activities and involvement. In time, the very being of the caregiver may quite unexpectedly have become engulfed by caregiving activities.

This gradual increase in caregiving is what occurred in our family as we became the unexpected and rather reluctant caregivers of my mother-in-law, Katharine. For us, the earliest sign of Katharine's decline was revealed quite suddenly to us when the electricity to her home was disconnected by the power company because she had neglected to pay her bill for several months. Until that time, we had no clue of her impending disease.

It was not as if we were neglecting Katharine. We visited each Christmas, spent two weeks with her every summer, and called her each weekend. Our weekly telephone conversations never hinted at any decline in her abilities. Of course, because we lived so far away, we were not in daily contact. Our career demands had brought us far from her Santa Cruz home many years before.

Despite our initial concerns about her lapse in bill paying, we managed to convince ourselves that Katharine's disorganized lifestyle was simply worsening. My husband thought it was his mother's eyesight that was failing. She was approaching eighty years old, and my optimistic husband was sure that she was having trouble seeing the figures and writing the checks. And I, as an accomplice in the earliest days of family denial, agreed to make an appointment for an eye exam for Katharine that July weekend. Katharine's eyes turned out to be fine. However, she had enormous difficulty trying to tell the opthamologist which of the letters on the many eye charts were better than the others. It seemed that she just could not choose. Katharine became frustrated and refused to cooperate in what she called the "nonsense" of the eye exam. She became agitated and very angry at the doctor because she thought he was tricking her. The doctor grew impatient, and during that appointment, I began to realize that Katharine's growing difficulties were much more serious than anyone else was willing to admit.

After many discussions that July weekend, I convinced my husband that Katharine's disorganization had now gotten to the point where she needed help with bill paying and finances. We both knew that Katharine had always had a relaxed attitude about organizing her home. An avid gardener and community volunteer, Katharine always had more important things to do than clean, and had never spent much time tidying up her house. Ever since I first met her more than twenty-five years earlier, she has had cleaning help each week. And, each week, as soon as the worker left, the clutter and messiness crept right back. I had always dismissed her disorganized house to her carefree attitude about life in general, but now her inability to organize and prioritize had reached a new level.

I was successful in convincing my husband that Katharine's monthly bills were probably becoming lost in the increasing clutter of her home. And, while refusing to admit that there was anything wrong with his mother, he reluctantly agreed that perhaps she did need help in organizing her finances. We finally decided that maybe it would be best to contact her telephone, electric, and insurance companies and ask them to send the monthly bills directly to our San Diego home so that we could take care of paying them. This was a significant concession for Dana. Always the sensitive and caring son, I know that he resisted taking over Katharine's bill paying because he was concerned that we might hurt her feelings if we even questioned her ability to continue handling the bills by herself.

While Dana and I told Katharine that we were going to help manage her bills, I was convinced at that point that she would not even notice that the bills had stopped coming to her Santa Cruz home. I knew that there was something seriously wrong. And while Katharine at first refused our help, we persisted, and she seemed to forget that she was even supposed to be receiving bills in the mail.

Looking back to when we began paying her bills that summer, I believe we can call that weekend the beginning of our family caregiving careers. More importantly, it was also the beginning of our family conflict over her symptoms and needs. Like many families, roles began to emerge even in the days before the actual caregiving seemed to occur. The Super-Caregiver role certainly emerged as I attempted to convince Dana and Katharine's other extended family members that there was something wrong. But, at the time, none of us recognized this as our early days of caregiving. Besides, Katharine seemed to be functioning on her own once we were helping her with her bills and finances. She was not driving, and she still kept up her garden club membership and church activities. Following that July weekend, Katharine never again mentioned anything to us about her bills. I am sure now that she never missed them. We returned to our San Diego home without fully comprehending that this was just the beginning of our journey through denial to caregiving.

What I did not realize then was that we were also setting up the dysfunctional coping style that would later make our caregiving so much more difficult during our first year with Katharine. Despite all of my years of research and teaching about the sociological implications of the aging of our population, I failed to recognize that we too were beginning a course of caregiving that would later threaten the functioning of our entire family.

The process that our family experienced mirrored closely the process of so many other family caregivers I have met in my teaching, research, and on our three-year caregiving journey. For many of us, caring for a spouse, a parent, or a parent-in-law with Alzheimer's disease is most often unexpected. It is a responsibility that most caregivers never sought, and sometimes may have even tried to avoid. Yet, it is a role that is being assumed by increasing numbers of children and spouses of Alzheimer's victims. However, families quickly realize that it carries tremendous costs.

For years, I have been teaching my gerontology students that family caregivers to Alzheimer's patients are more likely to suffer from stress and depression than any other group of caregivers. But in my own mind, I had always assumed that if the caregiver had enough resources, both financial and educational, that the caregiving could be managed without too much difficulty. On some level, I believe that I viewed the complaints of caregivers as evidence of weakness or disorganization. I was wrong. This arrogant attitude during our first caregiving year led me to think that because I have always been able to handle things so well, that I could surely handle taking care of sweet and easygoing Katharine.

What I learned and what I share here, is that arrogance can never play a role in caring for one with Alzheimer's disease. Even I, who foolishly prided myself on my ability to reach even the most recalcitrant students with just the right combination of educating and entertaining, cannot teach an advanced Alzheimer's patient a single new behavior. Our family experienced enormous stress. It is difficult to say whether the increased stress levels were due to the increasingly overwhelming demands resulting from the nature of the dementing illness itself, or if the stress arises because of the protracted nature of the caregiving. The awareness that the family commitment to caregiving can last anywhere from five to fifteen or more years can be an overwhelming thought for even the most committed caregiver.

Still, what I have found in our three years of caregiving is that there are some caregivers who have developed coping styles that have helped them reduce the stress and depression which can accompany family caregiving. I learned from them. In fact, I learned more from the family caregivers and those who support them through day-care centers and support groups than I ever learned in my Ph.D. courses in gerontology or in all of my academic research and reading.

Through our family caregiving experiences coupled with research and interaction with caregivers, I have identified three types of Alzheimer's caregivers. Caregivers within each type had developed coping styles and strategies that may have appeared initially to help, but, in time, these maladaptive coping styles may have actually caused additional problems and stress for the caregiver. I recognized myself in many of the caregivers' stories that I heard in support groups and in my research. Looking back to our earliest days of caregiving, I found myself first attempting the Super-Caregiver role.

Super-Caregivers are the perfectionists who think they can do it all. Super-Caregivers often seem to be working for an "A" in caregiving and in everything else they do. These ego-driven caregivers believe that they should be able to maintain full commitment to their careers, families, and their lives, while still assuming the primary caregiving duties for a demented family member. The Super-Caregiver may try to meet every need of the affected person, and refuse assistance or support from any source—because no one can provide the level of care that the Super-Caregiver can give. Failure is inevitable, because perfection is not possible when caring for a family member with Alzheimer's. Depression may then follow for the Super-Caregiver, as this ego-involved caregiver may begin to feel that he or she has failed to maintain the self-determined level of commitment to caregiving. At this point, Super-Caregivers also have a high risk of becoming Martyr-Caregivers when they realize that they can no longer maintain the perfection that they are attempting. They begin to relinquish other roles that may be interfering with their Super-Caregiving role. They may feel that they can indeed maintain the Super-Caregiving if they just let go of some of their other responsibilities, including careers, spouses, or perhaps even caring adequately for their own children. This is when they may move to the Martyr-Caregiving role.

Martyr-Caregivers have the tendency to sacrifice all other aspects of their lives to attend to the family member with Alzheimer's disease. Unlike the Super-Caregivers who attempt to do everything well, Martyr-Caregivers may withdraw from social contacts, leave their jobs, and later bemoan their fate. Sometimes, the Martyr-Caregiving may be initiated to compensate for some guilt that the caregiver may have about the one being cared for. The guilt may arise from failing to respond to the earlier symptoms quickly enough. Or it may evolve later in the caregiving career, from caregivers' feelings of failure that they were unable to provide perfect care for their loved one. Martyr-Caregivers may also arise from a formerly poor parent-child relationship for which the child is now trying to compensate. One Martyr-Caregiver I interviewed is still trying to make up for flunking out of college in the early seventies when her mother had paid for her education. For spouses, martyrdom can arise from formerly strained spousal relationships. If one member of the marital couple feels guilty about neglecting the impaired member during the marriage, becoming a martyr and sacrificing everything for the spouse may be a seductive way to try and make amends and lessen the guilt.

While any of these guilt inducing relationships can pull a caregiver toward becoming a martyr for their loved one, many family members become martyrs simply because they truly believe that it is the right thing to do. They often do not begin the caregiving with the intention of sacrificing their lives for the loved one. Instead, these quite noble caregivers may simply have a strong sense of filial or spousal responsibility and love for the impaired loved one. For many, the family bond is a very powerful one, with love as its foundation. It is when the love creates an overwhelming sense of responsibility that may cause the caregiver to give up his or her life to care for the affected family member.

Most Martyr-Caregivers find that they are even more stressed and depressed after giving up their outside jobs and social contacts. They may have more time to devote to caring for their loved one, but now that they no longer have outlets away from the caregiving, they are more depressed than ever. Following prolonged caregiving, desires to end the caregiving by any means often accompany the Martyr-Caregiving role. Thoughts of suicide, or thoughts of desiring the death of the impaired family member may occur when the depression turns to rage. There are stories in this book of family members who have actually attempted to hasten the death of their Alzheimer's afflicted loved one.

Reality-Based Caregivers are those who regard a diagnosis of Alzheimer's disease as a family and a community challenge, not simply an individual challenge or burden. Although they may have realistic fears and concerns about their limitations for the future, these Reality-Based Caregivers learn to draw upon the spiritual, emotional, and practical resources of their families and their communities as they attempt the journey of family caregiving.

It is my aim in this book to show readers how to become Reality-Based Caregivers. I do this first by recalling my own earliest days of caregiving, when I attempted the Super-Caregiving role. I provide examples of my own and others' caregiving experiences. I chronicle our disappointments over our inability to maintain the Super-Caregiving status, and my own perilous brush with Martyr-Caregiving, as I actually considered giving up a tenured professorship to fully assume the caregiving role. Throughout the book, I integrate research evidence with anecdotes from other families as they attempt to cope with caregiving by drawing upon each of the three caregiving roles.

The following pages will relate our journey from the apparent "perfection" of our lives before Katharine moved in with us, to the sometimes overwhelming challenges we faced in caring for her through the three years she lived in our home. I believe that our experiences will help other reluctant caregivers, especially the Super-Caregivers and Martyrs, to learn to take stock of their resources and draw from the help that is available to them as they begin a journey of caregiving to a loved one with Alzheimer's disease.

My main goal in *The Reluctant Caregivers* is to show family caregivers that through gaining insight into their motivations for caregiving and drawing from family and community support, they can move beyond maladaptive caregiving coping styles, to a rewarding Reality-Based Caregiving experience that benefits both the caregiver and the one receiving care.

Chapter 1

──────────── ❋ ────────────

Moving from Denial to Diagnosis

As members of the baby-boom generation, my husband and I should have expected the caregiving role. Baby boomers are approaching middle age in record numbers and should not be surprised that their parents and their spouses are aging. But, then again, as members of the "Peter Pan" generation of baby boomers who continue to deny our own aging, we all seem surprised when those around us have aged. A caregiving career is certainly not expected for the eternally young, former flower children of the sixties and seventies.

As one who teaches and writes about issues of the sociology of aging, I should certainly have expected the need for caregiving. I have been teaching my undergraduate sociology students about the implications of the graying of our population for more than a decade now. Indeed, the pattern of an increasing number and proportion of elderly persons in the U.S. population is not surprising to students of demography and gerontology. The aging of our population is entirely predictable from a theory of population change used by many demographers to explain the growth in a society's population. The theory is concerned with the relationship between birth rates, migration, and death rates, and the resulting effects on the age composition of the population. It helps us to understand and predict population trends like the current aging of our population.

This dramatic aging of the population creates an ever growing vulnerability to the diseases of old age like Alzheimer's. Although there are cases of early onset, the strongest predictor of Alzheimer's disease is advanced age. The average age of onset for Alzheimer's is from sixty-five to seventy-five years old. We now know that nearly half of all those over age eighty-five will show the dementing symptoms of Alzheimer's disease.

Whether caregivers expected the caregiving or not, we are documenting a dramatically increasing amount of care provided by the family for those afflicted with dementia related diseases like Alzheimer's. Today, nearly 70 percent of all dementia patients are cared for at home by family members. Study after study indicates that family caregiving is the most important factor in preventing or delaying the institutionalization of the patient. We know that the availability of family caregiving is the strongest predictor of whether the loved one will be institutionalized. We have found that the availability of a caregiver is even more important than the severity of the patient's impairment in predicting whether the loved one will live at home or in an institution. Yet, this family caregiving contribution is not without psychic and financial costs to the entire family. From the earliest signs of the disease to the final moments of the patient's life, family members will experience feelings of fear, frustration, helplessness, anger, sorrow, and sometimes depression and despair. Those involved in caring for the Alzheimer's patient fear not only what they are experiencing, but also what may come. Because of this fear, denial is an initial coping mechanism for many families. No one who has ever participated in a support group for caregivers will ever discount the power of the subconscious mechanism of denial that many family caregivers use in their early days of learning about the disease. Stories that caregivers tell about allowing their impaired loved one to continue driving a car point to the power of denial. My husband's interpretation of Katharine's inability to continue paying her own bills is certainly a good example of denial.

Denial can be useful in the earliest days of the illness because it may help family members ready themselves for what may come. However, if denial is prolonged, it can be dangerous by preventing the family from protecting the safety of the Alzheimer's patient or others with whom the patient may come into contact. To be fair to families who initially do not recognize the earliest symptoms of the Alzheimer's patient, we must acknowledge that denial may not always be the reason that family members fail to act early. During these early days of the emerging symptoms, it is often true that family members are at first unaware that their loved one is becoming seriously impaired. Often in the early stages of the disease, the signs are almost imperceptible. Unless the patient has insight into his or her disease and is willing to confide concerns about a failing memory, family members are often unaware of the memory impairment until it has advanced. At the early stages, many family members attempt to dismiss symptoms like forgetfulness and memory lapses as the normal part of aging.

In our family, I believe now that we never saw the earliest symptoms because my mother-in-law continued to look healthy and seemed to function well. Katharine had always been extremely independent since her husband died, nearly thirty years before. Since his death, Katharine had developed an extensive network of friends and activities. Because of her excellent health and high energy level, Katharine had maintained an active lifestyle of gardening, garden club meetings, church activities, shopping, and visiting with friends. It is possible that in these early days of her disease, Katharine's independence prevented her from confiding her fears of a failing memory. Whether it was her own denial or her stubborn independence that prevented her from sharing her concerns with us, we will never know.

There were unmistakable signs that we all failed to acknowledge. Like many families who are beginning to see behavioral changes in their loved ones, we know now that the symptoms were there, but we chose to dismiss them. For several reasons, we attributed these signs to Katharine's simply getting older. We joined the many other families who are watching their loved ones decline ever so slightly and saying nothing, because to admit that there might be something wrong with our beloved family member has serious consequences.

For many families, the most frightening consequences of an acknowledgment that there are behavioral changes in a family member is the concern that the person we care about may be becoming mentally ill. If family members begin making connections from the symptoms to a debilitating and eventually fatal disease like Alzheimer's, the realization is especially painful. There may be fears of loss of companionship and a loving relationship when the symptomatic loved one is a beloved spouse. For adult children, there may be fears of a loss of the parenting role of a loving parent. Or there may be fears of the unknown—not knowing what to do if there is, in fact, a diagnosis of Alzheimer's disease. The family members may know that if there is a diagnosis of Alzheimer's disease, then there must be a response from the family. Many family members fear that once they identify the problem, they will not know what to do to address the problem.

This process of denial may go on for months or more, until the loved one's behavior becomes too bizarre to be ignored. Sometimes, by the time the diagnosis is finally made, it may be too late. The Alzheimer's victim may have endangered his or her own life or the lives of others before family members acknowledge that there is indeed something wrong.

Denial is much more complex than family members realize. Because denial is an unconscious defense mechanism, most do not even realize that they are experiencing it. Even well-educated families miss important symptoms and opportunities to help the family member with early-stage Alzheimer's disease. In our family, our inability to acknowledge the earliest symptoms of Katharine's disease continued for nearly a year. And, by the end of that year, although Katharine continued to live alone, her behaviors became so increasingly bizarre that her Santa Cruz neighbors became alarmed.

Certainly, we should have seen the signs. Especially since I have spent the past ten years of my career teaching about the debilitating diseases of aging. Yet, I believe we all joined the countless other families who chose not to see what we later found were symptoms. The lapses in bill paying were early signs, but nothing could have prepared us for Katharine's behavior the following Christmas.

FORGETTING CHRISTMAS

We had just arrived at Katharine's Santa Cruz home for a Christmas visit and were beginning to unpack the car after our long drive up the California coast from San Diego. We had a trunk full of Christmas presents and holiday food for our visit. About five years earlier, I had begun doing most of the cooking at home for our holiday visits and bringing it to Katharine's home, because holiday planning and cooking had become too overwhelming for her. It had rained for most of the seven-hour drive from San Diego, and we all were tired.

Our son, Jonathan, had brought several of the bags from the trunk into the house and asked if we would mind if he watched television while we finished the unpacking. I knew he had been feeling deprived to have been "unplugged" during the long ride. But Jonathan returned quickly back outside to help us continue unloading our car. "Nothing is working in Nana's house," he pronounced. Apparently, when he tried to turn on the television set, Jonathan noticed that the cable box was blinking "call for service." He tried several of the lamps and none of them seemed to work.

We really didn't want to deal with appliance repair at that moment, but after investigating, we had to agree that Jonathan was right about the house—many of the appliances seemed to be broken, the television set plug was pulled out from the wall, the digital message on the microwave in the kitchen read "power failure," and the dishwasher was dismantled with the dish racks and soap dispenser piled precariously on the kitchen counter.

Like Jonathan, I knew that something was wrong in my mother-in-law's home. Actually, I had known at once, when we drove into the driveway and I noticed that Katharine's once lovingly tended rosebushes had begun to wither, but I didn't mention it to anyone else because I wanted the Christmas visit to be fun for our family. I didn't want my worrying to spoil the holiday, because it was the one time of year that our entire family would be together for a full week. Our daughter, Heidi, was completing her semester's work back at school. And Jonathan, like his father, always wants things to be nice, and for everyone to be happy. I was determined not to let my worries about Katharine spoil their Christmas.

Still, it was obvious that there was something "off," in addition to the appliances in Katharine's home. When we first arrived, I saw Katharine peering out the kitchen window, and I was shocked at her appearance. I had not seen her since the previous July, the weekend of the "power outage," and she looked like she had lost at least twenty pounds during the five months since our last visit. I waved hello and got out of the car quickly so that she could see us. Her face registered no recognition. It was obvious to me that she had no idea who we were until my husband came up to her kitchen window and said, "Hi, Mom!" Finally, she smiled her sweetest smile upon seeing Dana, her only child, and exclaimed, "What a nice surprise!"

At first we thought she was kidding, because we had just talked on the phone the night before when I told her when we would be arriving and what we would be bringing. But when we walked into the kitchen, we realized that she really was surprised by our arrival.

What struck Dana and me immediately was the realization that Katharine's house was a mess, not just disorganized and "lived in," as it had been since I first visited her home right after our marriage nearly twenty-five years before. Back then, as a young bride, I had loved everything about my new husband and had been actually impressed by Katharine's relaxed attitude about housekeeping. Having spent most of my life in Connecticut, I had always dismissed her messiness as a California relaxed eccentricity, while my husband joked about my own cleaning compulsion.

In contrast, Katharine always felt that she had better things to do than clean her house. Still, the mess that greeted us that December afternoon was well beyond even Katharine's California standards. There were clothes thrown on each of the chairs in the kitchen and piled on the living room chairs and sofa. There were dirty dishes overflowing the kitchen sink, because the dishwasher was obviously broken. She seemed to have forgotten how to operate many of the appliances, and apparently would pull the plug from the wall if she could not remember how to turn off appliances like the television. Most alarming of all, Katharine was dressed in a nightgown, even though it was the middle of the afternoon.

To Jonathan's observant eyes, there were none of the usual Christmas trappings. There were no decorations and none of the specially baked Christmas cookies and English plum pudding that Katharine had been baking since we first began spending Christmas together two decades ago. There was no wreath on the door that usually greeted us on these Christmas visits. It was clear that unless we moved quickly, there was not going to be any Christmas in that house. Katharine seemed to have forgotten Christmas!

We exchanged anxious glances as we brought our bags into the guest bedroom, but before we had time to talk about our concerns, we began to realize that the guest bedroom was even worse than the main portion of the house. The bedsheets were in a pile on the floor, as if Katharine had been abruptly called away in the middle of changing the bed and never returned to finish the job. All of the bureau drawers were open and the contents were hanging over the sides of each of the drawers, as if a burglar had just fled the scene after a frantic search for something valuable.

FAMILY DENIAL

During that visit, we began the first of many discussions that often became arguments about Katharine. This Christmas argument, like the arguments that would be replayed over and over during the next five months, began with my saying how "irresponsible" it was for us to allow her to live like that. Then, Dana would provide his usual dismissive response that it is not "as bad as you think," or his second and stronger option, "it's because you teach about aging that you see pathology everywhere." Or, the worst conversation stopper, "just because she doesn't keep her house as perfect as you keep ours, you think she's crazy." The discussions would end for a while.

It was not a pleasant Christmas for any of us. Our Christmas arguments set the pattern for what would later become a familiar dance that would continue for the next five months. I would lead with my concerns, and Dana would back away by reminding me that I was oversensitive to the symptoms of dementia. I usually would defer, because it was just easier than taking the real lead and actually doing something. It became easier to just let it go. And, I am ashamed to say that once we were back home in San Diego, I was again able to convince myself that Katharine was, after all, his mother and not mine. Besides, we made arrangements with the Santa Cruz Visiting Nurses to have an aide visit Katharine for four hours each day. The aide would help Katharine bathe and dress herself and would cook a meal for her. I reassured myself that the aide's daily visits would be enough to maintain Katharine in her own home. After a while, it became easier to convince myself that we were doing enough. And, like many families, we had help in our family denial.

ACCOMPLICES IN DENIAL

Denial in the earliest stages of a disease like Alzheimer's may be a way of protecting the impaired parent and the family members from the shock of the unwelcome news of the diagnosis. Early-stage denial may, in fact, help family members to control the way they finally receive the information about the disease. Denial buys family members time to adjust. In these early stages, denial can actually help loved ones to disengage from their feelings of fear for a while and distance themselves from the evolving symptoms of the disease. This can be a positive time of preparation, as long as it remains a short-term delaying mechanism.

Over time, however, the symptoms of Alzheimer's cannot be denied—no matter how hard the family members may have tried, and no matter how much help family members have received in confirming their denial. I have found in my conversations with families of Alzheimer's victims that there are often accomplices in the denial. A spouse who cannot live with the growing realization that his loved one is showing the unmistakable signs of growing forgetfulness or memory lapses, may enlist the aid of an adult child to help in the denial. This often happens, as the son or daughter may not want to hurt the feelings of the impaired parent, nor dash the hopes of the concerned parent. In these early days, the adult child may actually provide reassurances to both parents that these symptoms are just the signs of old age. The reverse is also often true, as the adult child may begin seeing the signs of the decline of a parent, yet the spouse of the impaired victim may refuse to acknowledge the impairment. This denial may persist despite the protestations of the adult child, who continues to attempt to convince the parent of the growing impairment. Often, out of respect, the adult children are unwilling to push the parent to initiate the diagnostic testing of the impaired parent, which would confirm the suspicions. In these cases, the family members act as accomplices in the denial.

There are other times when family denial can be so strong that if one family member dares to persist in pointing out symptoms and decline in the impaired family member, he or she is viewed negatively by the other family members. This conflict can set up a pattern that may be repeated throughout the course of the disease and the caregiving, and the recalcitrant family member may never be forgiven by other family members for bringing the bad news. Super-Caregivers often emerge in these early stages of denial by attempting to "take over" in pursuing a diagnosis. These determined family members may try to be helpful, because at this point, no one else is doing anything to address the growing problem of the impaired parent. Super-Caregivers may attempt to do this subtly at first, by providing reading material on Alzheimer's disease for the entire family. Later, when subtlety does not seem to be working, the Super-Caregiver may resort to continually pointing out symptoms of the impaired individual. Once this begins, these emerging Super-Caregivers have become the family "nags," because they are often pointing out the signs of the disease or reminding other family members that "we must do something." This cycle of symptom identification and reminding can continue indefinitely. But eventually, because of the progressive nature of the disease, the symptoms worsen sufficiently that other family members finally begin to acknowledge the problem, or worse, a life-threatening incident occurs which propels the family into action. Unfortunately, too often it is the latter, and the impaired individual begins presenting a danger to himself or others before the rest of the family notices.

Whatever the path toward diagnosis, the denial by the family and the ensuing targeting of the "messenger" of the disease is often replayed in the caregiving that evolves. Often, the family member who first identifies the symptoms and decline also becomes the one responsible for diagnosis, and increasingly, the primary caregiver. This assumption of the caregiving role can often be seen, in part, as a way to make up to the rest of the family for bringing them the bad news of Alzheimer's.

In other cases, ill-informed professionals may unwittingly become accomplices in maintaining the denial for the family. In our family, we had professional help in maintaining the denial of my mother-in-law's symptoms from her longtime family physician. During our July visit, she would tell us the same stories, and often repeat her sentences over and over. Although I realized during our visit that Katharine had many of the symptoms of the early-stage dementia characteristic of Alzheimer's, including memory lapses, forgetfulness, and repetitive speech, still, I chose to be convinced by my optimistic husband and Katharine's ill-informed Santa Cruz physician that I was imagining her symptoms. When her doctor told us that her symptoms were most likely due to her poor diet and anemia, we wanted to believe him. We never questioned whether her poor diet might have been secondary to her "forgetting" to eat for several days. On our last visit to her physician during the July weekend of Katharine's "power outage," her doctor told us not to worry and advised us to encourage Katharine to eat plenty of protein. He prescribed vitamin pills and ginkgo biloba because "it couldn't hurt."

While I had always had some doubts about this California physician's casual approach to medicine, on some level we all must have wanted to believe him. It is also likely that we may have underreported Katharine's symptoms to him. Katharine, appearing to have absolutely no insight into her symptoms, denied that there was anything wrong when he questioned her about her forgetfulness. She told the doctor that she was "tired of her family interfering in her business." In response, Katharine's doctor never administered any of the memory or orientation tests that we now realize we should have insisted upon at these early stages.

To be fair to this physician, he probably was filling our needs at the time also, because at this stage, our family was not ready for the diagnosis of Alzheimer's disease. The topic of Katharine's symptoms became the source of a cycle of conflict for us. Not wanting to maintain the role of the family "nag" in those early days of her disease, I joined the many family members who put their loved ones in great danger by allowing the pattern of denial to continue.

TWO MAJOR DANGERS OF DENIAL

While the very obvious danger that undiagnosed Alzheimer's patients present as they may continue to attempt risky behaviors like cooking alone in their homes, or simply crossing the street, there is another serious problem with family denial. This problem arises because of the missed opportunity for the undiagnosed Alzheimer's patient to participate in the drug therapies which may help to alleviate some of the symptoms. There are now new drugs available to early-stage Alzheimer's patients which hold the promise of actually altering the course of the disease. Two of the better-known drugs include Aricept (donepezil) and Cognex (tacrine). These drugs have shown promising results in delaying the progression of symptoms for early-stage Alzheimer's patients. In fact, the most recent research indicates that if prescribed early enough, and in a high enough dosage, both of these drugs may have the effect of actually significantly slowing the decline and damage to the brain caused by the disease, in addition to simply improving symptoms.

There are additional drugs which are currently being tested. However, a diagnosis in the early stages of the disease must precede the participation in all of these drug therapies. Families who continue their cycle of denial can actually cause their loved one great harm by delaying the identification of the disease until it has progressed to the point where drugs cannot help.

Unfortunately, our delay in diagnosis prevented my mother-in-law from benefiting from any of these drug therapies. Our inability to act until Katharine's behavior had become so bizarre that neighbors were noticing, probably exacerbated her symptoms and measurably shortened her life.

Looking back, we acknowledge that we should have acted earlier. We know now that there is nothing more important than a comprehensive assessment to help move the family from denial to definitive diagnosis and acceptance. This assessment must go far beyond a medical exam by a competent physician. The medical exam, coupled with a series of diagnostic tests supervised by a neurologist and a team of health care workers (including a psychiatrist and a social worker), is often the most effective way to move a family to action in responding to the growing needs of the Alzheimer's patient. Denial may continue to block family members from obtaining these diagnostic tests; too often it takes a catastrophic event to move families from denial.

MOVING TOWARD DIAGNOSIS

For our family, it was Katharine's neighbors' concerns that she was becoming a danger to herself that convinced us we needed to do something. Katharine was becoming lost in the neighborhood she had lived in for more than thirty years. In early spring of that most eventful year, we were notified by one of her neighbors that on several occasions in the middle of the night, Katharine would appear at her neighbors' doors to ask them where her house was. Always active and energetic, this was the first time that Katharine began exhibiting the wandering behavior, which later became one of the most challenging symptoms that she presented to us in our caregiving.

While slightly more common in male Alzheimer's patients than females, wandering behavior is often an attempt to "go home," even if the patient is at home. We have since learned that "going home" is often a metaphor for the Alzheimer's patient's desire to return to the past, when things made sense to them. This type of wandering can be very dangerous. But for many families, like ours, the danger that wandering can present is a major incentive to finally pursuing a definitive diagnosis.

With the family's realization of the seriousness of Katharine's wandering behavior, the diagnostic process was finally begun. It was also the time when the Super-Caregiving role emerged. Finding the best doctors, the most up-to-date diagnostic procedures, and the most comprehensive evaluation techniques is something that the Super-Caregiver thrives on.

We made the decision to move Katharine to our home in San Diego "for the summer" so that she could participate in the diagnostic procedures at the Medical School of the University of California, San Diego (UCSD). Having taught courses in the sociology of aging, I was impressed with the cutting-edge research that UCSD researchers and clinicians were doing in gerontology and Alzheimer's disease. I knew that their Alzheimer's evaluation procedures were not only the best in California, but were recently ranked among the top ten best evaluation centers in the country. I was familiar with the work of several of the UCSD health professionals, as they had visited our campus to present information about their gerontological research programs.

We told Katharine that we wanted her to visit with us for the summer to build up her strength. We assured her that the San Diego sunshine, good food, and company would make her feel better. Although Katharine denied that she was feeling badly, she had to acknowledge that she had lost weight. In fact, she seemed to be shrinking both in height and weight; even her shoe size had decreased. Katharine finally agreed to the short visit, and Dana brought her to our home on a sunny May day. We had no idea that we were assuming a burden that would quickly overwhelm our entire family.

Chapter 2

---------------------------- ❊ ----------------------------

Family Conflict and Caregiving

The protective cover of denial is removed from the family with the growing realization of the symptoms of Alzheimer's disease. Family members are no longer shielded from the difficult decisions that need to be made about the care of the impaired loved one, and, at this point, the family is left open and vulnerable to conflict about exactly what needs to be done. This can be one of the most difficult challenges in caring for the patient with Alzheimer's disease, because the conflict seems to emerge quite unexpectedly. In my conversations with family caregivers, I have found that family conflict over care plans and caregiving can create a severe source of stress, far beyond the actual tasks of caregiving.

Prolonged caregiving to a relative with Alzheimer's disease is a situation in which latent family strains are often activated, and conflict can displace prior family harmony. When this occurs, family members are likely to bear the emotional consequences. Family conflict can leave family members with severe emotional scars that may never heal. Having attended many support meetings where I heard stories of severe family conflict over caregiving dilemmas, I can recall feeling fortunate in some ways that my husband was Katharine's only son, and that we were the only available caregivers. My husband's father and brother had died several years before the onset of Katharine's illness, and although we often wished for someone to share the burden of the caregiving tasks, the family conflict that I witnessed made me actually appreciate our small family when decisions had to be made.

Because of the significant challenges presented to a family with Alzheimer's disease, family conflict seems to be almost inevitable. Although only one member of the family actually has the disease, the family itself actually becomes a "family with Alzheimer's disease," because the overwhelming caregiving demands upon family time and energy change family dynamics markedly. Formerly positive family relationships may actually be destroyed.

A recent, highly publicized case in the San Francisco Bay Area clearly illustrates the breakdown of a family with Alzheimer's disease.[1] The case involved the Klooster family, a longtime, highly respected Bay Area family. The patriarch, Dr. Gerald Klooster, formerly a successful and much-loved physician in the area, had been diagnosed with Alzheimer's disease and was being cared for at home by his wife. According to media reports, Dr. Klooster's wife was involved in a bitter custody battle with her adult son over the care of her husband. Published court reports and news stories both in print and on television news programs claimed that the adult son had found evidence that Mrs. Klooster had contacted the famous "doctor of death," Dr. Jack Kevorkian, to request assisted suicide for her husband. Mrs. Klooster had written several letters to Dr. Kevorkian, had purchased plane tickets to Michigan for herself and her husband, and had reserved a room for the two in a hotel adjacent to Kevorkian's home. Mrs. Klooster had also typed a letter to Kevorkian that she maintains was narrated by her husband, which stated that he did not want to continue living with the disease. It was signed with an "X," because Dr. Klooster was so impaired that he was no longer able to sign his own name.

Alarmed, the adult son left his own home in Michigan and flew out to the West Coast to attempt to dissuade his mother from her suicide plans for her husband. Apparently, discussions between the mother and son broke down, and Dr. Klooster's son actually kidnapped him to protect him from what he viewed as murder. Having accomplished the kidnapping, the son brought Dr. Klooster back to his own Michigan home.

The resulting court case generated great media interest. Family hostilities were broadcast each evening on the local television news. The national program *60 Minutes* taped a segment on the case. Each side made accusations that the other side did not have the impaired Dr. Klooster's best interests at heart. The Bay Area family members said that the Michigan son had never been involved in helping the rest of the family with caregiving, and therefore had no right to be involved. The bitterness of the family conflict was played out in the newspapers and before thousands of television viewers on the nightly news. One of the saddest parts of the story was the tragic attempt to interview the impaired Dr. Klooster on *60 Minutes*, when the reporter asked the visibly demented doctor where he wanted to live. He replied over and over, "I want to stay here in California." At the time, of course, Dr. Klooster was in Michigan, but had no idea where he was. Not surprisingly, both Dr. Klooster's son and wife interpreted the impaired man's response in the way that would support their own side of the case. Mrs. Klooster stated that Dr. Klooster's response was proof that her husband wanted to return to his California home. Dr. Klooster's son maintained that his father "knew" his home was now in Michigan. While the lower Michigan courts ordered that Dr. Klooster remain in the protective custody of his son's home in Michigan, appeals in both Michigan and California courts overturned that earlier decision, and the impaired father was again returned to the home of his wife in the Bay Area.

This sad story, unfortunately, does not end with Dr. Klooster's return to his California home. Several months later, the Associated Press reported that Dr. Klooster was rushed to the hospital, near death, having ingested a deadly combination of alcohol and sleeping pills.[2] While there were allegations again by the Michigan son that his impaired father certainly had help in taking the drugs, the event was ruled "accidental" by the California district attorney's office, and no one was charged in the case. Still, upon release from the hospital, Dr. Klooster was mandated by the California court to be moved to the Bay Area home of his adult daughter, Kristin. Media interviews with the daughter indicate that she supports her mother's decisions about her father's care and feels great animosity toward what she views as her brother's meddling in the caregiving. Throughout this case, there remains strong resentment within the family against the Super-Caregiving Michigan son, who tried to "take over" the care of his father. Because of concerns about another kidnapping by the son, Chip, neither Mrs. Klooster nor Dr. Klooster's custodial daughter will allow unsupervised contact between Dr. Klooster and his son.

While this case is indeed extreme, there are thousands of families who continue to experience severe conflict over Alzheimer's family caregiving. We know very little about the dynamics of this conflict, because few talk about it. In all of the books written about Alzheimer's disease and family caregiving, there is nothing about family conflict. A thorough search of the literature of the hundreds of academic studies on caregiving stress revealed only a handful of published studies that directly address the dimensions and consequences of family conflict in Alzheimer's caregiving families. It appears that family conflict does not interest most of the academic researchers involved in studying caregiving and the family dynamics of caregiving.

Still, anyone who cares for a loved one with Alzheimer's disease within an extended family context knows that family conflict can cause severe stress and depression for caregivers, well beyond the physical and emotional demands of the actual caregiving. The limited research findings that are available, and my conversations with caregivers, strongly suggest that family conflict is the problem most frequently cited by caregivers to Alzheimer's patients, over and above the actual caregiving tasks themselves.

SOURCES OF FAMILY CONFLICT AND CAREGIVING

In nearly every study of family conflict in Alzheimer's caregiving, it was of sufficient intensity to be considered a "serious problem" by the caregivers involved. When asked about the cause of the conflict, one answer emerged in nearly all of the published research—the conflict arose from the perception by one relative that another relative was not providing sufficient help in caring for the patient.

In one study by a researcher from Berkeley, California, the findings indicated that in more than 60 percent of the cases of family conflict, the cause of the conflict was directly related to the fact that the caregiver felt that other relatives were not doing their part in contributing to the care of the impaired family member.[3] This type of family conflict can be directly related to the adoption of the Martyr-Caregiver role by the primary caregiver. Suffering for the loved one while others in the family look on may feel noble at first, but the Martyr-Caregiving role eventually results in severe depression. And, because of the growing feelings of anger and resentment toward other family members, the caregiver becomes increasingly isolated.

In the research, the next frequently mentioned problem was, as the Klooster case so well documented, a relative criticizing what the primary caregiver was doing. For example, caregivers often report that relatives telephone and subtly, or sometimes not so subtly, suggest that the caregiver is providing insufficient care for the patient. One support group member claimed that her East Coast sisters would call and berate her for putting their mother into a day-care setting with, as they put it, "crazy people," just to get her out of the house. In response, this over-whelmed caregiver stated,

My sisters have no idea what it is like living day-to-day with a mother who thinks she is my child. She follows me around the house no matter what I am doing, even when I go into the bathroom to try and take a shower. She comes in and stands there and waits for me. I cannot get away from her, and because she is unable to dress herself or feed herself, I have to do everything for her. Day care is the only option I have. I would go crazy myself if I had to deal with her by myself around the house all day every day . . . My sisters just don't know, and I am angry at them for their attitudes about me. They should live in my house for a week with our mother. I guarantee that they would have her insti-tutionalized within the week. I get so angry.

Family disagreements over the long-term institutionalization of the impaired loved one constituted the third most frequently cited source of conflict. In these cases, the source of the conflict was disagreement over nursing home placement or even day-care plans. Part of the diffi-culty for the caregiver in this category of conflict was the implication that the disagreeing relatives would not provide further help to the pri-mary caregiver unless the caregiver complied in institutionalizing their loved one. This was especially true in the case of a spouse who is hesitant to place an impaired loved one, but feels pressure from the children to institutionalize the demented spouse. Additional types of conflict in-clude perceptions that one relative is taking advantage, by "stealing" money, furniture, clothing, or food from the demented relative; or, in other cases, relatives think that the caregiver is doing "too much" for the care recipient. One support group member said that her sister thinks she treats their father like a "child." A major source of conflict fo-cuses upon visiting; many caregivers feel that relatives do not visit the impaired family member enough.

It is also interesting to note that the caregivers most likely to experi-ence conflict were usually female, adult children of the Alzheimer's vic-tim. And "sisters" were the most frequently named source of conflict in the Berkeley study, which indicates that more than 35 percent of all caregivers named their sisters as the source of family conflict, 30 per-cent named their brothers, followed by a spouse (20%), a child (5%) or other parent (5%), or sibling-in-law (5%). Siblings or siblings-in-law thus constituted 70 percent of the relatives with whom the caregivers were experiencing conflict! Family conflict does indeed seem to be a sibling-related phenomenon.[4]

Many of these reported conflicts and resentments were quite strong. In addition to the Klooster case, there are several cases of family caregiving conflicts that have resulted in legal action. One woman described her siblings-in-law as "vultures," for only being interested in her father-in-law's money; another said that her family had "never been further apart until they began caregiving"; while a third cautioned: "Don't ever try to care for a parent because it will ruin your family relationships."[5] In a few of these family conflict cases, caregivers indicated that the family member had caused some problems in the past, so the current conflict was partly anticipated, although obviously not accepted. Still, in more than 80 percent of the family conflict cases, the conflict was recent and totally related to the caregiving. For example, the Berkeley study found that one caregiver said her sister had initially offered to care for her mother in exchange for being given the family house, but then tried to simply take the house and institutionalize the mother. This caregiver stated, "I don't understand my sister anymore, we used to be so close and now we don't even speak to each other. I get very upset."[6] Recalcitrant siblings seemed to cause particular problems, because caregivers felt that they had grown up together, knew each other well, seemed to share the same values, and should have been able to work things out. Still, spousal conflict should not be minimized.

SPOUSAL CONFLICT AND CAREGIVING

A recent caregiving memoir entitled *Looking After* by John Daniel beautifully captures the costs of caregiving for the marital couple. Daniel movingly describes the conflict that developed between he and his wife as he became the primary caregiver to his own Alzheimer's impaired mother in their home. In an attempt to enrich his mother's environment, he would provide stimulating experiences for her. He recounts bringing his mother outdoors to enjoy the evening sky:

There's not a lot of sky to see from our backyard, what with the tall birches and impinging rooflines of our house and our neighbors'. The stars we do see are only a few wan specks dulled by the diffused electric radiance of greater Portland. But the moon, riding high on clear nights or shining through thin overcast, sometimes with a coppery ring around it, the moon is something better. At some point in the fall of 1990, I started walking my mother outside at night to see it, especially when the moon was full or near full. It seemed a small thing I could do to get her off her bed for a while, to keep her in touch with the world of nature beyond the walls and roof of her circumscribed world.

It made me feel quite virtuous, of course. It quieted, at least temporarily, my nagging sense of guilt that I didn't spend enough time with her, that Marilyn and I were just boarding and feeding her until she died. A nice way of sharing something we didn't have to talk about, a nice way of saying good night.[7]

However, Daniel painfully recounts that in his efforts to enrich his impaired mother's environment, he began to realize that he was neglecting his wife:

What I didn't know at the time, and wasn't even close to knowing, was that Marilyn was upstairs sobbing into her journal as I walked my mother out and walked her back.[8]

The spousal conflict grew until Daniel's wife, Marilyn, finally confronted him with the fact that he was "consumed with caring for her." Daniel admits:

I could not see what Marilyn saw clearly, that the accumulation of those attentions had enveloped me and taken me over, so that between caring for my mother and trying to get my writing and teaching done, I had little time or temper for anything else, including my wife.

Without realizing it, Daniel was beginning to become a Martyr-Caregiver, giving up much of his personal life and his marriage for the cause of caregiving.

In most cases of spousal conflict over caregiving, there is serious disagreement over exactly who should be doing the caregiving. In our family, there were a number of reasons why I became the primary caregiver. Some of these were individual reasons, although as a sociologist, I must acknowledge that there are always cultural determinants. Whether dictated by culture, or by individual choice, I have always enjoyed taking care of others. And, in our marriage, as in most others, gender continues to play an important role in deciding who will do the caregiving. I will not say that my assumption of the caregiving was because of some sexist conspiracy on the part of my husband to assign the female-role stereotyped caregiving tasks to me. We never had that kind of traditional marriage, with rigidly defined gender roles. In fact, both of us have always had demanding careers which required sacrifices from each other to enable us to advance in our jobs. We both have made several geographical moves for our careers, and have always shared many of the child-rearing and household tasks.

Still, when it came to caregiving, my husband seemed unable and un-willing to assume the ever-expanding responsibilities, and I seemed to just "naturally" take them on. It is unclear whether he, like many baby-boom generation men, simply was not socialized to perform the personal care that Katharine required, or whether my early assumption of the Super-Caregiving role prevented him from providing the care.

Now that I am able to compare our family dynamics with those of so many others, I believe that socialization factors probably played the strongest role in the creation of the caregiving dynamics of our family and many others. While these newly liberated baby-boom men like my husband have become perfectly willing and able to help with child care, the reluctant male caregivers of today are simply unprepared for the intense personal care required in elder care. Even families without strict gender-role divisions may unexpectedly find that gender begins to play a stronger role than ever in determining who in the family becomes the primary caregiver.

One of the strongest themes I have heard over and over when interviewing family caregivers and their children is the continued acceptance that caregiving is a woman's role. While I might have expected this acceptance of traditional caregiving gender roles from women who had never worked outside the home, I was quite suprised to hear this from women with a history of substantial investment in careers outside the home. In conversations and support group meetings, women talked about feeling responsible not only for the personal care and nursing tasks, but also for the emotional well-being of the entire family. I found that I was just one of many caregiving women in the Super-Caregiving role.

While men may indeed love their impaired parents and may also have a strong sense of responsibility about their care, in general, when it comes to caregiving, men tend to do certain tasks reflecting the cultural assignment of gender-appropriate roles. Men like my husband assume the "male" tasks, including money management or bill paying. And, while men are major participants in making important decisions about caregiving, most of the caregiving families I have met continue to view the direct hands-on care of the elderly as a woman's role. John Daniel's book is so engaging because it shows a male caregiver actively involved in the physical and emotional caregiving of his mother, and it shows the toll on the marital relationship that the caregiving can take.

The sociological research consistently supports the dominant role that females play in caregiving. National caregiving data indicates that more than 73 percent of all family caregivers to the elderly are women. Of this group, 29 percent were adult daughters, 23 percent were wives, and 20 percent were other female relatives, including daughters-in-law. Husbands constitute about 13 percent of the caregiving population, sons make up 8 percent, and other male relatives, 7 percent. The absence of caregiving males provides little opportunity for a new generation of sons, like ours, to learn that it can indeed be acceptable for men to assume the direct caregiving tasks.[9]

Harvard philosophy professor Carol Gilligan writes about gender differences in caregiving, and asserts that the key difference between men and women stems from the disparate childhood experiences of girls and boys. Because of their socialization, girls tend to develop the inclination to sense other peoples' needs and feelings as their own. According to Gilligan, women judge themselves in terms of their ability to care. When boys see this female caregiving expertise, they internalize the role as being appropriate for females. And so it continues, even into the upcoming generations, despite what we had always thought were our best intentions to raise gender-neutral children.

To be fair, in our family I must also acknowledge my own role in taking on the responsibility of caregiving. Despite our dual-career family, caregiving as a female role was so deeply ingrained in my life that it did not even occur to me that Dana could have become a primary caregiver. When my grandmother's heart condition prevented her from living independently, my mother took care of her in our home. I had learned that women do the caring, just as Jonathan was learning now. The elder care that my mother did lasted only a few months, at the end of my grandmother's life. It seemed noble and good. I remember admiring my mother's loving care for her mother, and I remember thinking that it was an important thing to do—despite my mother's full-time teaching job.

This early socialization, coupled with the very pragmatic fact that my career allowed me to work at home, simply made me more available for the role. Unlike Dana, who works twelve-hour days in an office, I had always been fortunate to be able to write and prepare lectures at home. I had always structured my life to be available to my children, and now I was available for elder care also.

Like all Super-Caregivers, I became much better at the caregiving than anyone else in the family. Because I was spending the most time with Katharine, I became better than anyone else at understanding the "code" that her speech was becoming, and at interpreting her often bizarre behaviors. Within a few months of caregiving, I could almost predict her behaviors and be prepared for them. I knew when she was becoming tired or hungry. I also learned how to encourage her to eat, dress, and shower without an argument. No one else could do that—and, of course, no one else tried.

In contrast, Dana was always at a loss in trying to understand her. In the early days of caregiving, he felt that it was important to "correct" Katharine's mistakes. He had trouble with what he called the "dishonesty" of going along with Katharine's stories about visits from her mother or other deceased relatives. From my perspective, and from what I have learned from my own and others' experiences, it was better to "go along" with the things she would say. It was okay with me if she wanted to wait to eat dinner "until her mother arrived." I would simply tell one of the many white lies that I told her during those three caregiving years: that I would keep her mother's food warm in the kitchen or that her mother had already eaten and gone to bed. She was satisfied with these simple explanations and never pursued them any further. It made her happy for the moment to think that her mother was somewhere nearby, and when she was happy, everyone else could be happy too.

Dana, on the other hand, had trouble with what he viewed as this dishonesty. During the first year, he felt compelled to tell her that her mother was dead, or that she no longer lived in Santa Cruz. And each time he would tell her, Katharine would become angry and upset. She would actually mourn her mother's death every time he reminded her, because for Katharine, each time Dana would tell her, it was like hearing it for the first time. While he thought honesty was the moral response, he later learned that honesty with an advanced Alzheimer's patient can often be the cruel response.

By the end of the first caregiving year, Katharine no longer realized that Dana was her son. She no longer recognized Jonathan. Sometimes Katharine thought Dana was her brother, other times, she thought he was a stranger. By then, I had totally assumed the Super-Caregiver role, believing that I could not only be the best caregiver, but also continue a full commitment to the rest of my family and my career. While we had help at home during the weekdays while I was teaching, I was providing all of the caregiving in the evenings and during the entire weekend.

Too often, dysfunctional coping styles including Martyr-Caregiving and Super-Caregiving evolve from family conflict over caregiving. We have already seen how caregivers who feel that they have no help in the caregiving tasks often evolve into martyrdom. In essence, martyrdom is the tendency of the caregiver to sacrifice his/her life to attend to the patient full-time, all the time. This constant care is draining, both physically and mentally, and family conflict can actually close the door on the source of social support that might have been available to the martyred caregiver if open communication could have occurred earlier in the diagnosis and decision-making process. As a result of the conflict, the martyred caregiver now has no one to turn to for support, and anger and depression are common responses. In the worst cases, depression evolves into rage, and abuse may occur.

We can expect that as caregiving demands increase for the growing numbers of reluctant caregivers, family conflict will also increase dramatically. If recognized early enough, there are ways to avoid family conflict and dysfunctional caregiving coping styles.

WAYS TO AVOID CONFLICT AND MAKE FAMILY DECISIONS

Conflict will continue to characterize family caregiving unless these caregivers learn to communicate openly and honestly in the earliest days of the family diagnosis. While this is much easier said than accomplished, especially in families still characterized by denial and poor communication, there are some strategies. The first and most important strategy is to make a conscious effort to avoid the Super-Caregiving role. While the ego-driven caregiver may initially find satisfaction in being the "best" caregiver, the costs are too high. Too often, primary caregivers who complain about family members not being involved or not contributing to the care of the impaired family member have themselves to blame for setting up the cycle of isolated caregiving. These Super-Caregivers may have "taken over" the caregiving in the earliest days and appeared to other family members as already assuming the primary role. Only later do these ego-involved caregivers realize that Alzheimer's Super-Caregiving is impossible to maintain, but now that they are willing to ask for help, none is forthcoming because they may have already alienated other family members with their attitudes of superiority. Then, it is only a matter of time before the Super-Caregiver becomes the Martyr-Caregiver, and the cycle of anger, isolation, depression, and sometimes rage, is created.

How does one avoid the Super-Caregiver role? I found it almost impossible in our family in the earliest days, when others were unwilling to even admit that Katharine was seriously impaired. Without realizing it, I was setting myself up not only as the "family expert" on the disease, but also as the best caregiver. This was a serious mistake, because my superiority, and a host of gender issues, kept my husband from even trying to help in the care of his own mother.

I learned from this mistake, and have been helping other families avoid this serious error. I feel fortunate that I was finally able to recognize the dysfunctional Super-Caregiving coping style before it fully evolved into martyrdom. But, as the following chapters will show, Martyr-Caregiving is a short step from Super-Caregiving. I was beginning to become bitter and resentful. Fortunately, I recognized my anger before it evolved into something worse. Instead of depression, I had enough insight to be able to understand that I was at least partly to blame for taking over the burden of caregiving in my Super-Caregiving role. Eventually, my family began to share the burden, but that did not happen at all during the first caregiving year.

Communication is certainly key to setting up a family-friendly plan early in the caregiving journey. Instead of waiting until one of the family members begins feeling resentful about the burden of caregiving, plans must be explicitly stated, and all family members must come to some agreement. Caregivers now have some help in creating this plan from a new book entitled *Coping with Caregiving*, by Dr. R. E. Markin. Dr. Markin suggests that the family actually hold a meeting to fully discuss the diagnosis, the caregiving issues, and what options are available for the patient's care. While someone has to take charge of setting the agenda for the meeting, it does not necessarily mean that this person has to be responsible for every aspect of the family caregiving. Markin writes that "in the early days of caregiving, you must take charge of this family gathering and run it as formally as you possibly can."[10] He suggests that you create an agenda of the items to be covered and do not let the discussion wander too far afield. As in any family, there will likely be a diversity of personalities present, but the issues must be addressed in a rational and unified way. Markin advises that families should not "let any option go unconsidered, though sometimes the mere mention of the option of a nursing home or mental institution will bring abrupt and negative responses." If home care is the choice, decisions must be made about "whose home?" Once the site is chosen, each family member should be asked what he or she can do to help the primary caregiver. Some family members may be near enough to assist the primary caregiver in the home, attend to the patient a day or two each week, do the shopping, or help with the cooking or housework. Other family members, if they live too far to be of day-to-day help, may be able to provide financial support. If someone says that they can attend to the patient during the week, Markin suggests that the caregiver "get it in writing" by documenting the days and times. He also maintains that commitments of financial assistance be documented at the meeting.

Markin identifies an ideal agenda for the family meeting:[11]

Topics for the Meeting

The Patient's Current Condition

The Patient's Projected Condition

The Financial Situation—including Issues of Power of Attorney

The Care Options

Decision for Caregiving/Commitments from Others

While the formality of this meeting may be difficult for some families, and I know I would have a difficult time implementing some of the suggestions (especially the "getting it in writing" part), I do agree that it is necessary to have clear expectations for assistance from other family members. In many ways, I do feel fortunate that we did not have the hassles of family conflict to deal with. But, then again, we did not have access to the enormous potential for support that a loving extended family can provide in caregiving, when it is managed well.

When an extended family is involved, financial issues must be discussed as soon as possible, because these issues can create significant family conflict that can remain long after the caregiving ends. In addition, many caregiving decisions cannot be made without first addressing financial and medical issues for the impaired relative. Without durable power of attorney and a health care proxy, there can be no decisions made for the patient regarding his or her living arrangements, financial considerations, and access to health care.

POWER OF ATTORNEY AND HEALTH CARE PROXY

Because those with Alzheimer's disease eventually lose the ability to make decisions concerning their legal, medical, and financial status, family caregivers must address these issues as soon as possible after hearing the diagnosis. Once the patient's safety is assured, these financial and medical permission considerations should be the first issues that the family discusses. The ability of the family to be involved in decision making regarding financial and medical issues is yet another strong argument in favor of early diagnosis. It is so much easier for the family to complete these legal matters when the impaired member is still capable of sharing, to some extent, in this responsibility.

If the family delays, and the impaired person is no longer mentally competent, the transfer of power of attorney and health care proxy cannot be done by an attorney. Instead, the family must go through a lengthy and difficult process of petitioning the court for a guardianship of property (also called a conservatorship) and a guardianship of person. At a court hearing, a judge decides whether the person is mentally capable of handling his or her own property and financial affairs, which can be very painful for all involved. The process of conservatorship is portrayed in the classic film, *Miracle on 34th Street*. In this wonderful movie, a kindly gentleman with a fluffy white beard is convinced that he is Santa Claus and has an extremely difficult time proving it to the court in the adversarial competency hearing he endures.

Today, although courts are more familiar with Alzheimer's disease and a diagnosis from the patient's physician will usually be accepted as evidence, there is still a lengthy and difficult process for the family to endure. If the judge accepts the physician's diagnosis and rules that the person is indeed mentally incompetent, a guardian or conservator is assigned to care for the property under supervision of the court. The person named as conservator must file periodic reports to the court on the person's financial status.

Guardianship actions can be avoided, and the much simpler process of creating a durable power of attorney can be chosen if the person with Alzheimer's disease is in the early stages, and therefore still capable of sharing in the responsibility and signing the power of attorney. Power of attorney is greatly preferable to the competency hearings required for guardianship. However, family members must be careful to select the durable power of attorney instead of the simple power of attorney. Unlike the regular or simple power of attorney, which becomes void when the signer becomes mentally incompetent, the durable power of attorney gives the designated person the power to act and sign documents on behalf of the person with Alzheimer's disease when he or she becomes mentally incompetent.

The durable power of attorney is very important if the family needs to liquidate the assets of the impaired family member in order to provide care. For our family, the durable power of attorney allowed us to sell Katharine's Santa Cruz home and place the money from the sale into accounts to help pay for her monthly expenses, including the home health aides we began to hire to supplement our caregiving.

The health care proxy, or the power of attorney for health care, is equally as important as the durable power of attorney because it allows the impaired loved one to authorize a spouse, adult child, or close friend to make health care decisions when he or she becomes mentally incapacitated. The health care proxy should not be confused with a living will. The living will is necessary also, because it allows an individual to clearly state his or her wishes regarding the use of life-sustaining treatment. But the health care proxy goes well beyond a living will, because it can be used to make decisions about any and all health care measures. The health care proxy is needed to obtain medical care for the incapacitated loved one, or to even enroll the patient in a day-care program, a nursing home, or any health care institution.

OTHER FINANCIAL CONSIDERATIONS THAT LEAD TO FAMILY CONFLICT

Caring for an Alzheimer's patient is extremely costly. Financial considerations must be discussed as a family, because Alzheimer's disease can deplete a family's resources quickly. Because it is a chronic disease requiring long-term care, Medicare will not cover nursing care costs, home health aide costs, nor day-care costs. If the patient develops an acute injury or disease, Medicare will pay up to twenty days in a skilled nursing care facility and a portion of the daily rate for the next eighty days. However, the requirements for Medicare to pay for any health care costs are so rigorous that families should never count on Medicare for any assistance at all in the care of their loved one with Alzheimer's.

The husband of one of the women in our support group was hospitalized after he fell in their home. The physician recommended nursing home placement and rehabilitation following his release from the hospital. Unfortunately, the man had only spent one day in the acute-care hospital (this is another problem—hospitals are often in a great hurry to discharge the highly demanding Alzheimer's patients) prior to his transfer to the nursing home. This family learned too late that Medicare will not pay for nursing home costs unless the patient is transferred directly from the hospital to the nursing home after having spent at least three days in the hospital. The family had to pay more than three thousand dollars for the thirty-day nursing home costs, the ambulance to transport the man from the hospital to the nursing home, and for all of his medications in the nursing home.

Neither private health nor major medical insurance policies cover long-term home care or nursing home care. The exception to this is long-term care insurance coverage. While expensive, these policies are extremely helpful in paying for long-term care, day care, and institutionalization; however, these policies are unavailable to anyone with a diagnosis of Alzheimer's disease. Sometimes the person's life insurance policy may be a resource, if there is a long-term care rider to the policy. Again, however, these riders must be purchased before a person becomes incapacitated and diagnosed with Alzheimer's disease.

Medicaid is a federal program that is run and funded with federal and state tax dollars. It is only for the poor; however, it provides coverage for nursing home care, full-time home health care, and adult day care for those who are indigent. Generally, people become eligible for Medicaid only after they have depleted their own resources and assets and are below the federal poverty level. To qualify for Medicaid, the family home must be sold, and all resources must be depleted. There are exceptions to this requirement of full depletion if there is a surviving spouse who is living in the home. In the past, elderly couples would actually divorce in order to qualify the impaired member for Medicaid (or Title IXX) coverage to pay for nursing home costs. Fortunately, today we have the Medicare Catastrophic Coverage Act of 1988, which contains a spousal impoverishment clause, protecting the unimpaired spouse's financial resources when the patient requires confinement to a nursing home. The 1988 act allows the division of assets between the spouses and assures income for the well spouse still able to live in the community.

There has been fraud in the Medicaid system, however. Some families have tried to hide assets, or transfer assets of the Alzheimer's patient to other family members' names to qualify for state assistance in paying for nursing home care. It is considered a serious problem by state and federal agencies and is absolutely not advised, but there are lawyers who specialize in this type of asset management.

The fact that formerly law-abiding citizens would attempt this fraudulent practice is evidence that changes need to be made. Financial costs can be overwhelming and, when combined with the exhausting work of caregiving, it is understandable that caregivers feel burdened. In fact, financial considerations can indeed push some individuals to unspeakable acts.

FINANCIAL CONSIDERATIONS AND ELDER ABANDONMENT

There are families who, feeling desperate about the rising medical costs of the disease, have taken the immoral step of actually abandoning their Alzheimer's impaired family member. Precise numbers are not available, but researchers from the American College of Emergency

Physicians surveyed hospitals recently and concluded that up to seventy thousand elderly parents were abandoned each year by family members who were unable or unwilling to care for them any longer. "Granny dumping," as it has been called, was unheard of fifteen years ago. Now it has become a trend. A spokesman for the American Association of Retired Persons was quoted in the *New York Times* as stating that: "Not a day goes by when a hospital emergency room somewhere in America doesn't have a case where some elderly person has been abandoned, usually by the adult children."[12]

The most chilling example of the abandonment of an Alzheimer's patient occurred in Idaho. The *New York Times* reported:

Clutching a teddy bear as he stared out from a hospital bed near the dog racing track where he was abandoned, 82 year old John Kingery looked lost and helpless. But, the face, that of an elderly person who does not even know his own name and was left on society's doorstep could become a face of the future.

According to news reports, Mr. Kingery, who suffers from Alzheimer's disease, spent the last year and a half living in a nursing home in Portland, Oregon. The cost of his care was supplemented in part by Medicaid and Social Security checks. But, increasingly, Mr. Kingery's daughter was feeling squeezed by the financial demands made by Medicaid. Apparently, she became desperate. She checked her father out of the nursing home about ten hours before he was found near the restroom of a popular dog racing track in Post Falls, Idaho.

Holding a bag of adult diapers and a teddy bear, Mr. Kingery was found in his wheelchair, wearing bedroom slippers and a sweatshirt that read "Proud to be an American." The labels on his new clothing had been cut away, and all identifying markers on his wheelchair were removed in an effort to disguise where he had been. After being taken to a nearby hospital, Mr. Kingery spoke with detectives about his life of farming and his youth, but he did not know his name or where he had come from. He was incontinent and unable to walk. Mr. Kingery was finally identified, after administrators from his Oregon nursing home recognized him from a photo released to the national media.

It is not a crime in Idaho to abandon an elderly person who is dependent upon others for care, however, it is illegal to abandon a dog or a child in that state. Although many states have no laws making it illegal to abandon an adult, most states have laws that allow the state to intervene if the person has been judged incompetent and is not being properly cared for.

The fact that any adult child would abandon a parent with Alzheimer's disease is indicative of the desperation that some families face. While there may be no sympathy for the family member who could initiate such an immoral act of abandonment, these stories provide a frightening reminder of the measures that have been chosen by a very few, very desperate families with Alzheimer's disease.

NOTES

1. John Flesher, "Son Wins Custody of Father with Alzheimer's," *The Daily Iowan* (January 24, 1996): p.7A.

2. Martha Irvine, "Doctor with Alzheimer's Hospitalized After Drug Overdose," Associated Press (September 26, 1996): p. 2.

3. William Strawbridge and Margaret Wallhagen, "Impact of Family Conflict on Adult Child Caregivers," *The Gerontologist* 31 (1991): pp. 770–776.

4. Strawbridge and Wallhagen, "Impact of Family Conflict," p. 773.

5. Strawbridge and Wallhagen, "Impact of Family Conflict," p. 773.

6. Strawbridge and Wallhagen, "Impact of Family Conflict," p. 774.

7. John Daniel, *Looking After: A Son's Memoir* (Washington, DC: Counterpoint, 1996), p. 154.

8. Daniel, *Looking After,* p. 155.

9. Robyn Stone, Gail Cafferata, and Judith Strange, "Caregivers to the Frail Elderly: A National Profile," *The Gerontologist* 27 (1987): p. 620.

10. R. E. Markin, *Coping with Alzheimer's* (Seacaucus, NJ: Citadel Press, 1998), p. 27.

11. Markin, *Coping with Alzheimer's,* p. 29.

12. Timothy Eagen, "Robbed by Alzheimer's, A Man is Cast Away," *New York Times* (March 26, 1992): pp. 1B, 10B.

Chapter 3

──────────────── ❊ ────────────────

Creating a Safe Environment

"Just for the summer" . . . that was supposed to be the duration of our caregiving. In fact, we did not even originally define Katharine's visit that summer as an opportunity for us to provide caregiving. Instead, the plan was for Katharine to be with us just long enough to complete the diagnostic testing process. We thought that once the evaluation was completed, and a care plan developed for her own home, she would once again return to Santa Cruz with additional support. In anticipation of her return home, we had already inquired about home care services. We envisioned a friendly home health aide arriving at Katharine's Santa Cruz door each morning to help her with personal care, cooking, shopping, and light housekeeping.

We also anticipated that our lives would again return to the routines we had so enjoyed before Katharine's arrival. Yet, once we had the opportunity to see on a day-to-day basis how impaired she was, and how totally unable to live on her own, we knew we had to consider options other than her return to Santa Cruz. We realized that Katharine needed someone with her twenty-four hours a day! In this way, we joined so many other reluctant caregivers who are surprised to find themselves in the middle of a caregiving career that they had never before considered.

In our early caregiving days, we severely underestimated how much supervision Katharine would need. She moved in with us in late spring, and I thought that I could still leave her alone in the house for short periods of time. However, I found that I could not even go to the grocery store alone, because when I returned, she would be frantic with worry, forgetting completely that I had just left, even though I had reassured her that I would be "right back." I had to ask neighbors to come in and sit with her so that I could administer spring semester final exams to my students.

Even though she was requiring a lot more attention than we had anticipated, I knew that I was completing my teaching duties for the semester and would have, as my dear husband always reminds me, "plenty of time" to devote to the series of eight medical appointments necessary to complete Katharine's diagnostic assessment. And Dana was at least partly correct, because it was indeed becoming that wonderful time of year that all teachers love, when students begin to show signs of life, and teachers look forward to a summer of reading, writing, and preparing for the upcoming year.

Looking back on our innocent early caregiving days, I think of how much we all have learned since then. Spring used to be a self-satisfying time for me, because I used to allow myself to think that I may have played an important role in the students' blooming. It was this arrogant attitude that would later get us into trouble, as the Super-Caregiving role strongly emerged. It was arrogance during the first year that made us think that because we have always been able to handle life's challenges so well, that we could surely manage the care of a gentle woman like Katharine. Good-natured and generous, with never an unkind word about anyone or any thing, Katharine had been a loving mother-in-law during our entire twenty-five-year marriage. I often reminded myself that there probably was no one better to lead the caregiving than I. I had an office at home and did all of my writing there. In the earliest days of caregiving, I envisioned working in my home office during the day, as Katharine gardened or worked on the beautiful needlepoint she had always enjoyed. I anticipated that she and I would meet in the kitchen for lunch and breaks from our work. This fantasy lasted about a day.

The first week was a disaster. Katharine kept getting lost in our home. Knowing that Alzheimer's patients sometimes need visual cues, I created large signs directing her throughout the house. I bought poster board and drew huge black arrows directing her from the bedroom to the kitchen, and signs showing her where the bathroom was located. As a Super-Caregiver, I knew I could help her and our family live with the challenges she presented. By the end of the first month, we had signs everywhere in the house and in her bedroom, reading: "This is Katharine's room." But they meant little to Katharine; I had not realized that the Alzheimer's disease had so tangled her brain that she could no longer understand what the signs meant.

Still, the creative Super-Caregiver in me was undaunted. I decided that maybe she just needed a visual reminder of what was behind each of the doors. During month two, I began placing pictures on doors, thinking that if I put a picture of a glass of orange juice or milk on the refrigerator, she would know that "this was the place for milk and juice." I posted a picture of a bathroom on the outside of the bathroom door so she might be able to find the bathroom on her own. When that failed, we completely removed the bathroom door that adjoined her bedroom. Certainly, if Katharine could see into the bathroom at all times, she would realize where the bathroom was. She didn't.

Despite these early challenges, I knew that if anyone could manage caregiving, it should be me. I was a teacher of the sociology of aging, and therefore understood better than others exactly what was happening to Katharine's brain and behavior. I had taught about the physiological and psychological processes of dementia and had read and studied about many of the behavior management strategies of working with adults with dementia. Who better than I?

Most importantly, however, my husband and I agreed that we had to help Katharine. Strongly independent yet always willing to help others, Katharine had never asked for any help from us. Caring for her at this time seemed the least we could do. Guilt certainly played a role. After all, we were the same family members who had completely missed the earliest signs of her illness. We were the same family members who denied the symptoms far beyond the days that most others would have.

However, although theoretical knowledge may be helpful in setting up care plans, and self-confidence and self-assuredness are certainly important attributes for beginning a caregiving role, arrogance can never play a role in caring for an Alzheimer's disease patient. It is the most unbelievably, indescribably difficult job I have ever tried. Even I, who foolishly prided myself on my ability to reach even the most recalcitrant students, could not teach a new behavior to an advanced Alzheimer's patient like Katharine. Despite grand theories and behavior management techniques, I could not even help Katharine find her way around our own home!

Katharine needed help with every activity of daily life. She was never able to relearn her needlepoint skills, even though I kept buying easier and easier kits for her to practice on. She never was able to garden again, because she could not differentiate the flowers from the weeds. One morning, she pulled up all of our flowering impatiens before I realized that she was trying to help weed our garden.

Still, while we taught Katharine very little, she taught us something about ourselves. We had been seduced into believing that we could manage our lives without problems. We both had careers we loved, two generous and loving children, and a twenty-five-year marriage. Before Katharine arrived, I had often thought about how lucky we were. If it were a movie, the audience would have known that something bad was about to happen to the nauseatingly "perfect" family on the screen. We live in a beautiful old Victorian home in Mission Hills, San Diego. Even our city itself is often named in travel books as the city with the most "perfect" climate in the United States. Everything was perfect and we were proud of it all! Just as we began to be a little bit too proud of the perfection, it all changed.

Our home-based caregiving constantly reminded us that life cannot be perfect. Most people learn this earlier in their lives, because they face much more difficult challenges with far fewer resources than we had. I believe now that our arrogance about our perfect life in our perfect pale yellow Victorian home needed to be challenged. Katharine provided this challenge, because nothing is perfect when a loved one with Alzheimer's disease moves into your lives.

We quickly learned a lot about humility, patience, and compassion. Humility came at once—almost as soon as Katharine moved in with us, I found myself embarrassed by her behavior in public. During her first week, in an attempt to provide something to keep her busy, I invited Katharine to accompany me on a shopping trip to the Fashion Valley Mall, a nearby shopping center. She was enjoying the experience and all was going well until I became distracted in the shoe department at Macy's. Katharine had wandered over toward the women's clothing area. I heard some commotion and looked up in time to see Katharine standing in the middle of the department store without her blouse on. She had removed the blouse to try on some clothing, and was oblivious to the responses of the surprised shoppers. For me, it was the first of many humbling experiences.

Besides humility, Katharine taught us not to treasure material things too much. I learned not to take so much pride in our hardwood floors, oriental rugs, and antique furniture, because she unknowingly damaged much of this during her first weeks in our home. Not realizing how much trouble Katharine could get into, I had neglected to "Alzheimer's proof" our home by locking away cleaning supplies, and even things like hairspray, shampoo, and deodorant. I now look at the craggy-topped antique dresser that Katharine "polished" with the hair-spray she found tucked away in a bathroom closet, and begin to appreciate that she must have been trying to help me clean the house.

During those early caregiving days, it was a full-time job trying to keep Katharine safe and secure, and to keep her from doing too much more damage to our home. At that early point in our caregiving, our main focus was on safety. Until she arrived in our home, we had no idea how advanced her disease was, and how much trouble she could get into if left on her own. One morning, she tried to pour liquid Tide into her bowl of cereal. I had left her cereal on the breakfast bar and told her that the milk was in the refrigerator. I had also left the plastic container of detergent on top of the washing machine in the laundry alcove adjacent to the refrigerator. Both the door to the laundry room and the door to the refrigerator are white, and Katharine mistook the laundry room for the refrigerator. She knew she needed milk on the cereal, but no longer could differentiate a milk container from a liquid soap container. Worse, she could no longer differentiate a refrigerator from a laundry room.

We became increasingly frustrated by her behavior because we could not understand why she was doing the things she was doing. I knew about brain damage and brain cell destruction, but I was not prepared for the "misidentification" problems that accompanied this disease. So many other families have similar frustrations in trying to make sense of the seemingly bizarre behavior of their dementia-impaired loved one.

WHY DO THEY ACT THIS WAY?

In nearly every support group I have ever attended, the primary question of caregivers is, "Why do they act this way?" And, in the beginning, we began to have the same questions and very few answers. For Katharine, there was unmistakable evidence of memory loss and an obvious inability to focus upon tasks like paying bills, planning meals, and dressing properly. But we joined too many other families in missing the early symptoms of the disease because the signs are so subtle at the earliest stages. House keys are misplaced, names remain on the tip of the tongue too long and too often, the oven stays on after the meal is finished, and appointments are forgotten. All of these memory annoyances can be explained away for months and sometimes years, since the progression of the disease is often so slow.

If there is one definite statement we can make about Alzheimer's disease, it is that we simply do not know how quickly the disease will progress. Even with a diagnosis of probable Alzheimer's disease, the physicians cannot tell the family exactly when it may have started, or whether the patient will live for one year, five years, or even fifteen years! This uncertainty is because of the great variance in the onset of symptoms and the progression of the disease. Although the short-term memory loss and poor judgment eventually affect all Alzheimer's sufferers, there is great variation in the severity of the memory loss and in how quickly the disease progresses. This progression is directly related to the damage that is occurring in the brain.

The fundamental nature of the disease is the progressive degeneration and loss of vast numbers of nerve cells in those portions of the brain's cortex that are associated with the so-called higher functions, such as memory, learning, and judgment. Severe loss of these intellectual functions interferes with the person's daily activities and may cause the affected individual to behave peculiarly and show impaired judgment. When an older person loses the ability to remember, think, and act with good judgment, that person is suffering from senile dementia. Dementia is really a group of diseases which can be caused by Alzheimer's, stroke, depression, poor nutrition, diabetes, or a number of other maladies. But Alzheimer's disease is by far the most common cause of dementia, and the damage that it does to the brain is far more destructive. For example, while a stroke does its damage all at once, Alzheimer's gradually does more and more damage each day. This means that different cognitive abilities are damaged unevenly, and the person will be able to do some things but not others.

When brain damage is uneven, the person will do things that simply do not make sense to us. When the person does something especially odd or unexplainable, like pouring Tide on cereal instead of milk, it means that some part of the brain has failed to do its job. For example, one of the caregivers in our support group told us how her husband had become obsessed with the junk mail that arrived at their home each day. He believed that he needed to attend to each piece of the mail. While he still had the capacity to read his mail, and he still knew that the mail could be important to read, his brain was no longer capable of filtering out the things to which he did not need to attend. His poor wife was bewildered, because her demented husband felt that he had to respond to each solicitation to refinance their home, or use coupons at local restaurants, or have the house painted (even though they had a brick house). She worried that he appeared to be studying the many mail solicitations for carpet cleaning, window replacements, and home financing. She said that he was "thoroughly consumed by an ad offering a low-cost vaccination clinic for pets," and clipped the ad, even though they had never owned a pet.

We had similar experiences with Katharine. We found that we had to turn off the television news programs each evening once Katharine moved in with us, because she was unable to separate herself from the reports of muggings, fires, homicides, and robberies reported nightly on our San Diego local news stations. Katharine was convinced that the violent events would happen to her or to our family and became upset. It was apparent that she, like many middle-stage Alzheimer's patients, no longer had that "instant" filtering mechanism that most of us have which helps us determine whether something needs our attention. While most of us pick up our mail and throw the junk mail solicitations into the trash, early- and middle-stage Alzheimer's patients can become a marketer's dream, because they feel that they need to attend and respond to everything they read. This can be especially dangerous if the Alzheimer's patient has access to the cable shopping channels and still has the ability to dial the phone and use a credit card. The impaired judgment, coupled with this lack of filtering abilities, can result in financial ruin for the family. It is not unusual to hear of an early- or middle-stage Alzheimer's patient emptying out the family's bank account and having no idea where the money has gone.

The severity and nature of the individual's dementia at any given time is directly proportional to the number and location of brain cells that have been affected. As Dr. Sherwin Nuland so clearly points out in his book, *How We Die*, the decrease in the nerve cell population is in itself sufficient to explain the memory loss and cognitive disabilities. Still, there is another factor that seems to play a role in creating the severe dementia associated with Alzheimer's, namely, a marked decrease in acetylcholine, the chemical used by these brain cells to transmit messages.[1]

In order to function, different parts of the brain cells and neurons must communicate with each other. This depends upon electrical impulses that are the product of neurochemical interactions. The chemical that leads to communication between the nerve cells is known as a neurotransmitter. Acetylcholine is one of the most important neurotransmitters. The brain uses chemical raw materials to manufacture acetylcholine within the cells of the brain. The acetylcholine then transmits its messages to other brain cells. When the message is received, these cells break down the used acetylcholine. Because Alzheimer's disease sufferers have less than 50 percent of the acetylcholine that nonsufferers have, effective neural connections simply are not being made.

Further, when groups of nerve endings scattered throughout the brain cortex degenerate, the resulting areas of degenerated neural material disrupts the passage of electrochemical signals between the cells. Plaques and neurofibrillary tangles can then develop. The greater the number of neuritic plaques and tangles, the more disturbed is the intellectual functioning and memory.

Because of the great variation in nerve cell damage, tangles, and brain shrinkage resulting from the disease, there is also great variation in the symptoms from patient to patient, and sometimes from day to day in the same patient! After days of making no sense, an Alzheimer's patient may have a lucid interval and be able to carry on a conversation that appears in every way to be normal. This happened frequently during our first caregiving year, and in many ways made the caregiving even more difficult, since we could never really predict how Katharine would respond to any situation. One day, Katharine was unable to dress herself or brush her own teeth. The next day, she amazingly would not only dress herself, but would even correctly make her own bed and figure out a way to unlock the complex locks on the front door that we had installed to prevent her midnight wanderings!

One of the most intriguing symptoms was what I used to call Katharine's "data merge." She would appear to combine or collapse information from various sources in her mind and merge them into a whole—even though they were completely unrelated. For example, Katharine persisted in thinking that our daughter, Heidi, was a nun! This would be especially amusing to those readers who know Heidi, because although she is a kind and wonderful person, she is definitely not a nun. But each time I would mention Heidi's name, Katharine would immediately ask how things in the convent were. On one of Heidi's visits home on a semester break from school, she had a date with an old friend. Katharine mentioned several times how nice it was that "they were finally allowing nuns to date these days." We finally figured out that Katharine had merged Heidi's "files" with those of her niece, Jane who has been a nun for several years, and of whom Katharine was always very fond. In this case, Jane was merged with Heidi. I, too, became merged with Katharine's aunt and sometimes even her mother. And, in Katharine's mind, Dana took on the identity of her brothers Cliff and Dan, and sometimes, her father. Some of these merges made sense, but other times, it was as if a disk had crashed and files were merged in a bizarre combination. Naming of items were also problematic. The first of many times she misplaced her eyeglasses in our home, she asked us if we knew where the "windows" were. Because it was early in the caregiving,

I thought she was just confused about our windows and proceeded to point out all the double-hung windows in her room! She, of course, became frustrated, and I, in turn, became exasperated. Eventually, we learned that words had very different meanings. Shoes were called boats, and spoons were called shovels. Katharine most often named items by their function instead of their appropriate name. This is common in Alzheimer's patients, and families need to be creative in interpreting the functional names for items.

The brain damage itself can account for some of the variation we used to see in Katharine's day-to-day functioning and abilities. Researchers believe it is possible that damaged nerve cells which fail most of the time do work occasionally. It is also possible that less-damaged or undamaged areas can intermittently take over temporarily. Katharine's unevenness in ability often reminded us of an antique lamp we have that needs rewiring. Sometimes the lamp will switch on when we turn the switch, other times, we have to turn the switch ever so slightly to make it click on. Still other times, it turns itself on and off because of the faulty connection.

Alzheimer's patients often seem to be making faulty connections. Although each individual is different in his or her rate of disease progression, there are, in fact, several identifiable phases of the illness, each bringing its own set of symptoms and caregiving challenges.

Like most other families, once we acknowledged that Katharine was suffering from dementia, we wanted answers about how quickly the disease would progress, or how far the disease had already progressed, and finally began the diagnostic process. Again, we underestimated the severity of Katharine's impairment.

THE DIAGNOSTIC PROCESS

Katharine began the outpatient evaluation process at the University of California, San Diego Senior Only Care Clinic (SOCARE), during that first summer in our home. The UCSD diagnostic process follows the protocol recommended by the National Institute of Health and is similar to the one used by Alzheimer's diagnostic facilities throughout the country. It includes a medical evaluation, psychological assessment, neuropsychopathic testing, neurological examination, and a social work assessment.

As the first step in UCSD's evaluation process, Katharine received an initial medical examination which included a medical history, a family history, and a thorough medical exam. Because of her inability to recall medical and family history, I provided the information, and a physician administered an exam. The physician also administered a three-part test of orientation, which included the following, questions: Do you know who you are?, Do you know where you are?, and, Do you know what date or year it is? Katharine knew her name, but had not a clue about where she was, how she had gotten to the clinic, or what year it was. When he asked where she was, she responded, "here."

The medical evaluation also identified a gait instability. Katharine's ability to walk had become severely impaired. Many Alzheimer's patients have a wide-based gait like Katharine's, and use tiny steps and a forward thrust of their heads as they walk. The experienced neurological clinicians at UCSD detected motor system abnormalities upon initially encountering Katharine in the waiting room. Her stooped posture, slowness in standing, and difficulty in beginning to walk were clearly visible to the neurologist.

In addition to the medical and neurological exams, several laboratory tests were done, including a blood count and thyroid function test to rule out other causes for the dementia and neurological problems. This really is the purpose of the evaluation process; ruling out other causes like depression, diabetes, or other medical causes helps physicians make the diagnosis. At present there is no "definitive" diagnosis for Alzheimer's disease, therefore, when all other causes are ruled out, Alzheimer's is the final diagnosis.

A CT scan of Katharine's head showed central and peripheral atrophy of her brain. The scan also showed what they termed "bilateral lentiform nucleus calcifications, most likely degenerative, and a small area of deep white matter disease adjacent to the tip of the anterior horn of the left lateral ventrical portion of Katharine's brain." All are suggestive of Alzheimer's, but not definitive.

Based upon her medical history and exam, together with Katharine's poor response to the three important orientation questions and her impaired gait, the physician identified "an insidious onset of a gradual progressive and now severe dementia, in need of a full evaluation to determine the cause." The full evaluation process began the following week with an appointment at UCSD for a bio-behavioral evaluation and a full mental status exam.

The biobehavioral evaluation is important to determine whether the demented patient is depressed. Depression can cause symptoms similar to dementia, and it can make an existing dementia worse. Katharine was interviewed by a UCSD psychiatrist who noted that she had dementia, but ruled out depression as the cause.

The mental status screening is meant to determine how severely the dementia has progressed and to help plan a course of treatment. The cognitive status exam consisted of tests of Katharine's level of consciousness, ability to concentrate, orientation, existing fund of information, ability to learn new information, and judgment, as well as her short- and long-term memory. UCSD administers many of the same mental status screening tests that are available at diagnostic centers throughout the country. Usually, the first tests include those that assess patient orientation, and include questions about the patient's name, age, and occupation, as well as identification of the year, season, date, day, and month. The patient's fund of information is evaluated by asking for the names of the United States president and vice president, and the state governor. Further inquiries are often made about current events and the significance of these events, as assessed from current information in newspapers and other media sources, such as television. Typical questions concern the activities of the president, upcoming elections, and well-described conflicts throughout the world.

The ability to learn new information is assessed by giving the patient the names of three common objects, such as a golf ball, a sailboat, and an automobile. The evaluator names each object one second apart, and asks the patient to repeat all three objects immediately. Short-term memory is tested by repeating the test of the three objects until the patient is able to name all three, then waiting five minutes and asking the patient again to name the three objects. Long-term memory is evaluated by asking for the patient's birth date, date of marriage, date of military service if appropriate, and the dates of major events, including world wars and the dates of Christmas and other holidays. Testing the ability to calculate requires asking the patient to subtract 7 from 100 serially, and to perform simple addition, subtraction, multiplication, and division.

Language function is evaluated by noting the patient's capacity to form full sentences, understand and follow three-step commands, identify right and left sides, name fingers correctly, read simple sentences, and write sentences. The patient's ability to draw and copy diagrams of simple objects like a rectangle, square, cube, and clock face is also determined.

Judgment is finally assessed with what is called the "letter and fire test." The patient is first asked, "What would you do if you found a stamped, addressed, sealed envelope on the street?" Then the patient is asked, "What would you do if you were in a crowded theater and you saw a fire?" Other means of evaluating judgment and intellectual function include tests of similarity. For example, the patient is asked, "How is a bicycle similar to an automobile?" Or, "What is the meaning of the proverb, 'people who live in glass houses should not throw stones'?" Not surprisingly, Katharine performed poorly on all these tests. In fact, at the start of her medical exam, when the nurse asked her to "hop up on the scale," Katharine tried to hop. Alzheimer's patients take everything literally!

The above-described quantitative tests of mental status function are typical of those offered at most diagnostic centers. They include the Blessed Information and Orientation Tests, the Goldfarb-Kahn, the Ward-Kahn, the Mini-Mental State Exam, and the Dementia Rating Scale. Katharine achieved the following dismal scores: Blessed, 9 correct out of 33 items; Goldfarb-Kahn, 3 correct out of 10 items; Ward-Kahn, 3 correct out of 10; Mini-Mental State, 14 out of a possible 30; and on the Dementia Rating Scale, Katharine achieved a score of 99 correct out of a possible 144.

While we were saddened by the low scores, we had some relief, because finally we had documentation of what we had known. Still, none of us were prepared for the severity of the impairment. Because of her significantly low scores, Katharine was pronounced too severely demented to even attend the Alzheimer's Association "Morning Out" day-care activities. She had scored only nine correct out of thirty-three items on the Blessed, and she would have needed to score more than twenty-one to participate in the early-stage Alzheimer's Association activities. It was also at this screening that Katharine's dementia was deemed too far advanced to make her eligible for participation in the early-stage Alzheimer's drug therapies. We finally became most aware of the damage done by delaying the diagnosis.

These mental status exams were painful for both Katharine and for us. For Katharine, it was frustrating to be unable to answer so many of the questions posed. Although she still seemed to have no insight into her disease, she was perceptive enough to know that she was failing in these tests. We were embarrassed and sad that we had delayed so long before we had confirmed our fears. The UCSD nurse practitioner who had administered the mental status exams said, not unkindly, that "it is unusual for a family like yours to allow the dementia to progress so far without a diagnosis." She was right, and we were properly humiliated.

We knew then that Katharine would never be able to return to her home. And we knew that we had to make changes in our home to accommodate her. We began by "Alzheimer's proofing" the house.

"ALZHEIMER'S PROOFING" THE HOUSE

We quickly learned that our home had to be "Alzheimer's proofed" in much the same way we had "baby proofed" the house with the birth of each of our children. We also realized that it is much more difficult anticipating what an agile Alzheimer's patient can do, and how he or she processes information. An Alzheimer's patient is tall enough and strong enough to open doors, windows, cabinets, and closets. The Alzheimer's patient can turn on the oven, the washing machine, the dishwasher and all of the water faucets—sometimes all at the same time!

We became Home Depot's best customers in their locks and latches department. Before we installed locks on our closet doors, Katharine's favorite nighttime activity was emptying the first-floor closets and packing our clothes while we slept upstairs. The first night she was in our home, I got up in the morning and found that she had emptied our cedar closet and had packed everything, including my favorite cashmere camel hair coat. It really would not have been much of a problem, if she had not also smashed bananas, cookies, and hot dog rolls into the same suitcase.

During these early days, Katharine was very busy indeed. She slept in short naps during the day, and seemed to be awake most of the night. This is typical of Alzheimer's patients, as they are often unable to achieve the deep REM sleep that so benefits the rest of us. To fill her nighttime hours, packing was her favorite activity. Even when we removed the suitcases from the downstairs closets, Katharine still managed to pack several clothing items into shoe boxes, Kleenex boxes, and even jewelry boxes. Each evening after dinner, she would go into her bedroom and return carrying her slippers, her toothbrush, and a Kleenex box stuffed with her nightgown. She would then announce to all of us that she had enjoyed her dinner with us, but she had to "go up home now." After about a week, I stopped trying to talk her out of it and simply said that I would bring her later. Within a few minutes, she would forget and would eventually go to bed for a little while.

Anticipating her behaviors, we became so creative with installing locks everywhere in our house that our son began calling our home "The Rock." We joked when we unlocked one area of the house to enter another that we were "entering Cell Block C." We installed wrought iron security bars on the ground-floor windows in Katharine's bedroom and bathroom, because she had already tried to "escape." Once we had the home secured with locks, alarms, and bars designed to keep

Katharine inside, we began to worry about planning our escape routes in case of a fire.

While each Alzheimer's patient is different in his or her rate of disease progression, nearly all caregivers will be confronted with many of the same behaviors I have just described. Wandering and obsessive behaviors like packing and pacing are common, as are hoarding and hiding. While we never had to deal with clinging behaviors, or the combativeness and anger that can make caregiving a nightmare, these too are behaviors related to the disease process. Caregivers, especially reluctant caregivers, need to be ready for these behaviors by creating a safe and secure environment for the impaired loved one and for the rest of the family.

Regardless of what stage of Alzheimer's disease the patient is in when the decision is made for in-home care, it is never too early to begin anticipating the need for making the environment safer. It is helpful to begin with some general guidelines for safety, and then proceed to assess each room in the home for safety concerns.

General Guidelines

1. Install security locks on all exterior windows and doors. Remove locks from inside rooms so that the impaired loved one cannot lock him/herself in the room and deny access to the caregiver.
2. Keep medications out of reach or locked away.
3. Remove scatter rugs. Tack down edges of carpet. A dark-colored scatter rug looks like a black hole to an Alzheimer's patient. In fact, some creative caregivers have placed a dark-colored rug on the floor to prevent the patient from wandering further.
4. Keep all appliances in a locked closet, including electric knives, irons, hair dryers, and sewing machines.
5. Remove poisonous plants, including holly berry plants (because Alzheimer's patients may try to eat the berries).
6. Purchase an alarm system that rings when a door to the outside is opened. There are inexpensive systems that can be easily installed. Alarms are safer in the event of a fire than dead-bolt locks that need a key to open them, although we found that we preferred the dead bolts at night instead of being awakened every few hours by the security alarms.

In addition to these general guidelines, there are room-specific guidelines that are helpful:

The Kitchen

1. Remove refrigerator magnets that look like food items. We had a plastic magnet that looked like a chocolate-covered candy, and Katharine tried to eat it.
2. Remove the knobs from the stove. We have a gas stove, and finally removed the knobs so that Katharine would not turn them on each time she passed by.
3. Install child-proof latches on cabinets, drawers, and water faucets.
4. Turn off the water source for the washing machine and unplug the clothes dryer each time you use it. There are some things you cannot control in this area. Katharine once removed the clothes dryer lint screen and I was unable to find it for weeks. Eventually, I found it lying propped against a window in the house. Katharine had obviously misidentified it as a window screen.

The Bathroom

1. Remove all soaps, shampoos, hairsprays, deodorants, nail files, scissors, and dryers, and keep them in a locked closet.
2. Replace glass shower doors with a shower curtain, because Alzheimer's patients have trouble seeing the glass.
3. Purchase a locking device for the toilet tank so that an impaired patient cannot disassemble the plumbing in the tank. We became very good customers of a local plumbing company because Katharine was often trying to "repair" our fixtures. She often complained that the toilet was not working properly. We were pleased to find that there are indeed ways to lock the tank itself.
4. Turn off the water source to the sink and tub when not in use so that the Alzheimer's patient cannot overflow them.
5. Consider covering the mirrors in the bathroom or bedroom if the reflection becomes too disturbing to the patient. At the middle and later stages of the disease, the Alzheimer's patient no longer recognizes him/herself, and can become frightened by the "person" in the mirror. We never covered the mirrors, since Katharine seemed to enjoy smiling at and talking with the "person" in the mirror. In fact, she would always say hello and smile at the reflection in the mirror wherever she was. The first time we noticed this was on the mirrored elevator in her doctor's office building. She got on the elevator and began a conversation with herself in the mirror. Because she had such a pleasant and engaging face, she always enjoyed what sociologists might call the ultimate "looking-glass self."

The Bedroom

1. Try to arrange a first-floor bedroom if at all possible. Alzheimer's patients are not adept at going up and down stairs. In some ways this helped us, because we really only had to worry about securing the downstairs of our home.

2. Unless you are willing to straighten out the closets each day, it is absolutely necessary to purchase a lock for the closet doors. Rifling through clothes closets and cabinets is a common behavior. In my visits to residential Alzheimer's facilities, I noticed that each patient's room contained a locked clothes closet to assist the already overburdened staff.

3. Unless the Alzheimer's patient is completely bed-bound, resist the temptation to purchase a hospital bed. Hospital beds with rails may seem like a good idea to keep the impaired individual in bed, but the railings provide a climbing site for most early- and middle-stage Alzheimer's patients. This can be dangerous. A better alternative for the patient who frequently falls out of bed is to place the mattress and box spring directly on the floor. We removed the frame from Katharine's bed and placed the mattress and box spring on the floor in her room.

Although these safety and planning lists may seem excessive, we found that we had to plan for almost every occurrence with Katharine. Always an active and energetic person, she had never been content to sit and read or watch television. Before her illness, Katharine loved to garden, go for long walks, go shopping, and visit with friends. And even though she was now incapable of pursuing any of these behaviors in a rational way, she thought she was continuing them. She remained "busy" and in constant motion at all times, and thus needed to be supervised or in a safe environment at all times.

In addition to these safety concerns, there were other behavioral management strategies that we needed to learn, when Katharine began to have what seemed like hallucinations, but were in reality more like serious misidentifications. For example, Katharine's first-floor bedroom was located in an area of the house where water from our second-floor plumbing passed through the pipes adjacent to her room. Every time she heard the water going through the pipes, Katharine was sure that she was becoming drenched. She convinced herself that water was coming through the windows and wetting everything in her room. It made her extremely agitated, no matter how many times we tried to reassure her that it was the water passing through the pipes. After a while, it became easier to simply agree with her, and tape newspapers onto the panes of the window in her bedroom to "keep the water from coming in." There were many times when we simply went along with her perceptions, even though there was no basis in reality.

For example, Katharine was convinced that her eyes had developed a constant blinking movement. Of course, she was making them blink, but had no consciousness of doing so. We convinced her that the doctor ordered some special "anti-blink" eye drops, and would pretend to put Visine into her eyes whenever she would complain. Our pretense of simply holding the eye drops over each eye would immediately stop the blinking and the complaining for a while. After a few months, she moved on to other behaviors.

We became extremely creative in dealing with all of the misidentifications Katharine presented by never minimizing them, and always attending to them. When she was convinced that the lint in her shoe was not lint, but moving bugs, I immediately took the shoes out of the room and brought a different pair in for her until I cleaned the lint out of the old pair. We always took her seriously, because to her, these were indeed frightening occurrences.

One thing we were grateful for was that Katharine's wandering dramatically decreased by the second year. Not all families are that fortunate and to help them, the Alzheimer's Association has developed the Safe Return Program. The patient is given a bracelet similar to the Medic-Alert bracelets. The Safe Return bracelet has a phone number to call, which then matches up the registration number on the bracelet with that of their files. Therefore, if the patient becomes lost, the registry number on the bracelet will help reunite the patient with his or her family. Without the Safe Return bracelet, wandering Alzheimer's patients are in danger of becoming arrested, or worse. When we first purchased our Safe Return bracelet for Katharine, she kept taking it off until I used "crazy glue" on the clasp. The bracelet then stayed in place for more than two years.

The Alzheimer's Association suggests that the family keep recent pictures of the impaired person, along with an accurate description of such characteristics as hair color, height, weight, and other identifiers, as this information can increase the chances that the person will be found quickly. They also suggest keeping a clothing item that the patient has worn in a plastic bag so that it can be used if dogs are used in the search process. I remember being frightened when I read that direction; however, the reality is that too often Alzheimer's patients do indeed become lost. Dr. Klooster, the San Francisco physician previously discussed, became lost for nearly two days in the earlier stage of his illness. This is not uncommon. We often hear stories of "missing persons" on the evening news in San Diego, and they are often described as "elderly and confused." Wandering is a serious problem, and although we found ways to restrict Katharine without her feeling "confined," we must admit that we were not always ahead of her. Many of our solutions were responses to mistakes or near-accidents. And there were many times when we attempted to end the lesson by relinquishing the caregiving to someone else.

Throughout the first caregiving year, I visited more than twenty nursing homes and Alzheimer's residential programs throughout San Diego County looking for the "perfect" placement for Katharine. Because of the overwhelming caregiving demands and safety concerns, most professionals will advise placement in a secured facility for the Alzheimer's patient following the diagnostic process. At our medical consultation following Katharine's assessment, the well-meaning physician advised that we "should begin looking at once for a placement for Katharine because her behavior will worsen gradually to the point where the rewards of caregiving will disappear." It was hard not to smile at that statement; I remember wondering what "rewards" he might have been referring to. At that point, during those first months, we certainly were not finding any rewards. Looking back now, I recognize that on some level we might have been feeling a degree of self-satisfaction that we were providing a safe, secure, and loving environment, and that we were fulfilling our family obligation. We might have been feeling some reprieve from the guilt that we had felt during the early diagnostic days. But both of these emotions were related more to ego satisfaction than to anything else.

Still in the Super-Caregiving mode in those early days, we said nothing about our overwhelming concerns to the kind clinicians gathered for our family consultation. While we appreciated the candor of these university-based professionals, we decided to at least consider the possibility that we could keep Katharine at home. However, we realized that we could not keep both her and the rest of the family safe without some help. I needed to return to teaching in the fall, and our son was beginning to feel, most severely, the parenting deficit that caregiving had caused. Tied to the house and to Katharine for most of the summer, we were unable to take a vacation or even make our usual summer trips to the San Diego Zoo or La Jolla Shores that we had always enjoyed. The constant caregiving began to take a toll on all of us. Heidi was away at school on the East Coast, so she was relatively unaffected by the disruption to our family life, but Jonathan suffered.

We decided to hire live-in help. I was hopeful that once we did, our problems would lessen. However, we learned that although financial resources can buy some respite, caregiving to an Alzheimer's patient is not a job you can usually "give away." In fact, in many ways, our caregiving became even more complex. The presence of live-in help actually created many more problems, because of the growing disruption in our family life. We found, like other families, that children seem to suffer the most—too often they are the silent victims of the caregiving.

NOTE

1. Sherwin Nuland, *How We Die: Reflections on Life's Final Chapter* (New York: Random House, 1995), pp. 89–117.

Chapter 4

---------------- ❋ ----------------

Children Who Care

In many of the books about caregiving, the primary caregiver is often called the "hidden victim" of Alzheimer's disease, because this physical effort often results in exhaustion, sleeplessness, or even physical injury. Because of our family's experiences and those of other family caregivers I met, I found that the emotional stress experienced by young children and teenagers who live in the same home with an impaired parent or grandparent, makes them the real "hidden victims" of Alzheimer's disease.

Children and teenagers living with an Alzheimer's disease victim are often dealing with complex emotions. In my conversations with them, I have found that nearly all of these children and teenagers feel fear. They are afraid of what their impaired relative may do, and even more afraid that they or their parents will also become Alzheimer's victims. This fear is often coupled with anger, resentment, tension, and anxiety.

ANGER AND RESENTMENT IN CAREGIVING CHILDREN

Anger is a common response from older children in caregiving families. This is especially true for teenagers, who may feel resentful that their homes are no longer their own. They may feel a loss of privacy, or that they can no longer invite friends over to their homes because they fear the embarrassment that the impaired family member may cause for them. They may be unable to listen to music or watch the television programs that they enjoy, because it may be upsetting to the impaired grandparent. They may be angry with their caregiving parents for devoting so much time and energy to the grandparent instead of them. They may be resentful that family vacations had to be postponed or cancelled. Or, these children may simply be angry about the tremendous changes that have occurred in their homes and in their lives.

One caregiving mother found that her eleven-year-old daughter wanted to eat dinner alone in her room, away from the rest of the family, because she said she was "so disgusted by her impaired grandparent's table manners." This daughter's anger became especially strong toward her father because the family was now caring for "his mother." This is not unusual. In fact, there were a few instances in our own family, when our sensitive and loving son, Jonathan, reminded his father that it was indeed "his" mother that was disrupting our lives.

Anger and resentment can also arise for teenagers when they feel embarrassed by the behavior of the impaired relative. There are several cases of this described in Elaine Brody's book, entitled *Women in the Middle: The Parent-Care Years.* In one case, Brody describes the teenagers in the caregiving Carter family:

The teenage children could not bring friends home because the behavior of their grandmother was disruptive and embarrassing. A granddaughter begged for a high school graduation party. She had never had a party before. Mrs. Carter agreed and planned to send her mother to another daughter's home for the evening. But, the mother became ill and was unable to leave. There was no party. The granddaughter is now receiving psychiatric care.[1]

The chaotic Carter situation was characterized by disorder and conflict between the extraordinarily difficult elderly mother and everyone else in the family, especially the children. Many more families in Brody's study experienced similar stress. Children of Super-Caregivers and Martyr-Caregivers seem to suffer even more, because they may begin to feel abandoned by the caregiver's over-involvement with the impaired family member.

Caregiving parents are often surprised to find that their children's anger is directed at them and not the Alzheimer's victim. This is not unusual, especially for older children and teenagers, who have learned that the victims of Alzheimer's cannot control their behavior. Anger may be felt by the child and is often directed at one or both of the parents as the cause of the family problems.

It is becoming increasingly clear that children who grow up in dysfunctional caregiving families share a negative view of aging and elderly individuals in general. Indeed, they are more likely to view all elderly persons as a burden and as less competent than the nonelderly. As a result, these children are less likely to develop healthy relationships with even unimpaired elderly people. Because of their negative childhood and young adulthood caregiving experiences, these children may be unwilling to assume caregiving duties for their own parents in the future.

Diane Beach, Ph.D., one of the very few researchers exploring the effects of Alzheimer's caregiving on children, has found that the stress that accompanied caregiving had a negative impact on the caregiving childrens' relationship with both elders and other family members. Specifically, Beach found that these children talked about the significant decrease or altogether elimination of "normal" family discourse, the vying for attention from the primary caregiver, and the confrontation of outright violent behavior on the patient's part. One child said, "It takes away from our time together and whenever we're all together in that situation sometimes we end up getting frustrated with one another."[2] Another child lamented the loss of her mother and her grandmother: "It's frustrating for me because I guess I'm still a child and want my mom to take care of me and that sort of thing, and she doesn't have time to do that. And, I'm in a better position to take care of myself than my grandmother, so I'll be expected to just take care of things on my own for a while."[3] Another child worried about his father's Alzheimer's disease-related anger: "He had been angry for years even before he was diagnosed. We just thought he had an extremely bad temper and now it's frustration. You can tell it's frustration. He gets mad at me, but he gets mad at my mom more."[4] One child sadly talked about the indignity that her father suffered because of his Alzheimer's disease: "There is really nothing you can do, you know. Before I left, he was becoming incontinent. He couldn't get to the bathroom in time and he would have wet areas on his pants and that would bother me, but I wouldn't really be embarrassed for myself. I was more embarrassed for him because I know he wouldn't want to be seen in public like that."[5] It is not unusual for children to feel this ambivalence and this strong sense of loss and sadness. This very sadness characterized our family.

SADNESS

Our son was completing fourth grade when his grandmother moved into our home. Always kind and sensitive, Jonathan's life changed dramatically during that first year. He never really complained about his grandmother, and never confided in us about his feelings about her living with us. Instead, Jonathan wrote about his feelings in a story he created for a school assignment the following fall. The story was so sad that we became concerned.

Jonathan's fifth-grade creative writing assignment was to create a fictional story about a boy who faces a significant challenge and overcomes it. Jon titled his story *The Rock* and created a main character named "Reggie." His "fictional" story began:

Reggie had just ended the biggest day of fourth grade, the class trip to Sacramento. It was on May 19th and the whole class flew from their hometown of San Diego to visit the capital in Sacramento. Reggie thought it was the best day of his life until he got home and saw his Nana with Alzheimer's sitting in his living room. That was the exact moment that an evil force took over his life.

Chapter 2 of Jonathan's book presents the "challenge":

Now that Reggie's Nana moved in, a lot of problems have come about. For example, the family now needed a live-in helper. Carla, the helper, always said if she didn't like the dinner. So Reggie's Mom would always prepare things that she liked. But, Carla didn't like Reggie's favorite foods like spaghetti or pizza. Carla liked steak and tacos. So, you can see, Carla was almost as big a problem as Reggie's Nana.

Another problem was that Reggie's Mom had to miss special events at Reggie's school like the fifth grade Explorer's Day. The Nana was always complaining about things. One day she wanted a haircut and when Reggie's Mom didn't take her right away, the Nana found a scissors and cut all her hair off. After that, she looked like a boy with a really bad haircut.

Reggie's house had locks everywhere because his Nana would always try to go home to New York even though she didn't live there for a lot of years. There were so many locks everywhere in Reggie's house that it was like that movie about Alcatraz. That is why Reggie called his house *The Rock*.

Jonathan's book provided us with examples of the stress that "Reggie" experienced, and the ambivalence that children often feel:

Even though some solutions have been found, Reggie sometimes has a lot of anger and stress. Usually he thinks it is his Nana's fault, and in many cases this is true. Also, sometimes he thinks he should get a little more attention. But, don't get him wrong, he doesn't want the whole world to know about Reggie, he just wants a little more attention. Reggie sometimes has to come up with something on his own to relieve his stress so he goes out to the driveway to shoot some baskets. But, one day when Reggie was outside shooting baskets, Carla let her grandchildren visit and go upstairs and play with Reggie's toys and video games. Reggie's Mom was nice and forgave them. Reggie never did.

Jonathan's epilogue was all the more heartbreaking, because although he tells us that "years later, all the practicing paid off and Reggie reached his goal and became an NBA player," we readers sadly learn that "Reggie's Mom has become a real expert on Alzheimer's disease and now takes care of Reggie's dad who just came down with Alzheimer's."

When we read Jon's book, we were struck by the description of events that we thought he had barely noticed. We were even more shocked by the overwhelming sadness that flowed through the writing. There was sadness evident in his feelings about the loss of his grandmother, but there was much more sadness about the loss of his own parents, who were now so engulfed in their caregiving tasks that "Reggie" seemed to be getting lost. His book showed us that he recognized the sadness in all of our lives, yet in "real life" Jonathan responded quietly and sympathetically by never complaining and frequently offering to help.

Even when his grandmother created embarrassing situations for him, Jonathan never seemed to become angry or frustrated with her. During those first few weeks in our home, before we realized exactly how impaired she was, Katharine provided a source of embarrassment many times. During the first week, we made the mistake of bringing Katharine to the Spring Concert at Jonathan's school. Jonathan was performing with his fourth grade class. Katharine and I sat near the back of the crowded auditorium. The concert had barely begun when she stood up and announced that it was time to leave. I whispered quietly, "in a few minutes," and took her hand to help her sit down again. Within two or three minutes, Katharine stood up again. I whispered again, to ask her to sit down. We did this standing up/sitting down routine three more times before I gave up and led her out of the school auditorium and brought her home.

When I returned to the concert, having missed Jonathan's performance, the only concern he voiced was that I had missed the concert. He never complained that his grandmother's behavior caused him any embarrassment, although I know it did. We never brought Katharine to another school event, but this incident was significant because it created what Jonathan seemed to construct as a three-year moratorium on inviting his school friends to our home. We know that he was embarrassed by her often odd behavior and did not want to expose his friends to her. We also know that Jonathan hated to go out to public places when it included Katharine. He would often decline an invitation to go out to dinner if the invitation also included his grandmother. Still, he never complained. It became obvious that unlike many caregiving children, Jonathan had pushed aside his fears and directed his anger and frustration inward. In many ways, this can be much more damaging and could have led to a childhood depression had we not realized what was happening. We feel fortunate that Jonathan was able to articulate his feelings in a creative writing assignment. We were finally able to talk with Jonathan about his own feelings, and while it never disappeared, his sadness and fears were eased.

While Jonathan was indeed a "hidden victim" of the disease, most of the children of caregivers seem to outwardly suffer more from emotions like fear, frustration, anger, and resentment. Fear is especially common. The conclusion of Jonathan's story about "Reggie" clearly showed his fears that his own father might become a victim of the disease.

FEAR AS A COMMON RESPONSE FROM CHILDREN WHO CARE

Even very young children have complex feelings which they may or may not express about the illness and the caregiving roles in the family. Children may be afraid of the behaviors of the impaired loved one. These fears often have a legitimate basis. For example, one caregiving parent described her seven-year-old child's fearful reaction to her impaired grandfather's nighttime wandering behavior. During the night, her grandfather would wake and become confused and disoriented in the house. He often would wander throughout the house and sometimes would end up roaming around in the child's bedroom. This became terrifying for the child, who then began wanting to sleep with her parents. It took sleeping medication for the grandfather and several months of reassurance before the child would again sleep in her own bedroom.

In a few Alzheimer's caregiving families, there is violence and aggression when the impaired patient feels frustrated or angry. Having witnessed the violent and explosive tantrums of their demented relative, children in these families have very real fears of being injured themselves. Some Alzheimer's patients exhibit very frightening behaviors, and children should never be exposed to this threat of violence. Certainly, placement outside the home is necessary in these cases, if behavioral management strategies or medication to control the aggressive Alzheimer's behaviors are not effective.

Despite these examples of reality-based fears of the symptoms of the disease, many children's fears are of the disease itself. For Jonathan, the fear that his father may eventually become a victim of the disease was disguised in his book. Living with the fear of Alzheimer's disease can indeed bring a sense of sadness into the life of any child or adult. Fear is a stressor, because it can detract from everyday life. A fearful child often becomes an anxiety ridden, neurotic adult, incapable of living life to its fullest. For this reason, fears must be addressed.

To address his fears about "catching" Alzheimer's, we provided Jonathan with some very basic information about genetics and the inheritability of the disease. He was studying some very elementary-level genetics in his fifth-grade science class, and already had a rudimentary understanding of the role of chromosomes and genes. By selective information sharing, we were able to assure Jonathan that the late-onset form of Alzheimer's disease that his grandmother had is much less likely to be passed on to future generations than the more virulent, early-onset form of the disease. Should children begin asking the kinds of questions that Jonathan began to ask indirectly through his writing, parents can find information about the inheritability of Alzheimer's disease in chapter 7. While most children would be unable to read and understand some of the more complex genetic information, parents may be able to interpret some of the more basic and less threatening information about the genetic risks to help ease the fears of their anxious preadolescent or teenage children.

Of course, none of this information should be even discussed with children, unless parents believe that the child is becoming concerned about their parents' or their own risk factors. Many children do not even know about inheritability factors, and they probably should not be told unless they begin asking questions. In many families, discussion about family genetics or other instances of possible Alzheimer's disease in previous generations is overheard by the children. This "genetic gossip" can be a source of great concern for children. In our family, we have learned never to assume that we know what our children are thinking. We know now that we needed to initiate these discussions, because many children like Jonathan do not want to cause an additional burden for their parents. Jonathan would never have disclosed his concerns without our originating the discussion. For him, the fears became sadness. For other children, fears may lead to anger and resentment.

During our earliest days of caregiving, Jonathan often felt angry with his father, because he realized that I was doing most of the caregiving and that I no longer had the same amount of free time to spend with him. I seldom attended his school basketball games and increasingly was missing important school events. We tried to address Jonathan's parenting deficit as soon as we realized that he was indeed feeling lonely. Dana began to assume many more of the parenting tasks that I was missing. He began coaching Jonathan's YMCA basketball team. He taught him to play golf. Within a short time, Dana and Jonathan would spend much of the weekend together going to Jonathan's basketball games, the movies, the zoo, or to ball games. Golf games could last five or six hours on a weekend. Jonathan seemed happier, and Dana was certainly enjoying the time with his son. I remember feeling that I should be grateful that Jonathan was now so engaged with his father, but instead, I found myself feeling tremendous resentment that Dana was having all the fun and I was doing all the work!

Martyrdom was fast approaching. I felt angry and resentful about being at home alone with Katharine all day on Saturdays and Sundays, while Dana and Jonathan were involved in their activities. Even though I never lost my patience and understanding with Katharine, and I know I still was a loving mother to Jonathan, I was not a pleasant person to be around. For me, it was the beginning of what I now recognize as the "Martyr phase" of caregiving. It was the most troubling period of our entire family caregiving career.

CHILDREN AND MARTYR-CAREGIVING

A martyr is one who willingly suffers on behalf of a cause. Saints are often called to martyrdom because they are willing to suffer and die for the higher purpose. Caregivers, on the other hand, can evolve into martyrs when they become overinvolved in the cause of caregiving; their martyrdom results in growing isolation and alienation from others. A cycle is begun—as the caregiver becomes more of a martyr, people move further and further away, increasing the isolation and alienation.

Martyrdom can also evolve from an overwhelming sense of responsibility combined with an almost masochistic need to suffer for some imagined or real grievance. And, while the causes for the martyrdom may differ, the effects are similar. For children and other family members who are living with a martyr, the sense of abandonment that grows out of the caregiving can deprive a child of his or her childhood, and can destroy loving relationships between spouses and siblings.

Families can disintegrate when a caregiver moves into martyrdom, because no one can quarrel with the noble sacrifice that the martyr is making. These Martyr-Caregivers take Super-Caregiving a step further, and are willing to give up everything for the "cause" of caregiving. While appearing selfless, these caregivers often forgo friendships, careers, social activities, and sometimes other family members so that they can be totally devoted to the caregiving cause. Everyone else in the family suffers when a family moves into martyrdom. This is especially painful for children.

Martyr-Caregiving causes children to choose one of two coping responses. Some children appear to rise to the occasion and become *Super-Helpmates* to their martyred caregiving family. While these children may appear to be coping well by providing support, this Super-Helpmate role also carries costs. A missed childhood is one casualty, as the young child assumes too many responsibilities while missing out on the activities of childhood.

A far larger number of children of Martyr-Caregivers find the caregiving family dynamics so painful that they withdraw completely from the dysfunctional family system and choose to escape.

Escapee-Children are those who are able to withdraw from the martyrdom that is characterizing their dysfunctional family caregiving. While more common in college-age and young adult children of caregivers, there are also young caregiving children who psychically opt out of the martyred family caregiving circle. These children may retreat to their bedrooms or to friends' homes because they no longer feel that their home belongs to them. These young escapees may find refuge in reading, television, or computer games. As part of his escape, Jonathan located several sports-related web sites on the Internet. While Jonathan's weekends were filled with basketball and golf games away from home, each weekday evening after dinner was spent "away" in his room doing homework. His grades were excellent, and Jonathan found a way to escape while still remaining home.

On the other hand, young adult children of martyrs are able to escape both physically and emotionally from the dysfunctional caregiving family. Although it may be unspoken, they realize that they too are expected to sacrifice their lives for the impaired family member. Often they refuse, but their refusal carries a heavy price.

Julie Hildon, author of *The Bad Daughter*, is an example of a young adult escapee from a dysfunctional caregiving family. Hildon's mother's early-onset Alzheimer's disease coupled with her martyred aunt's expectations for her, pushed her to move far away from the family and become involved in a life that was more rewarding. Hildon was remarkably successful in escaping. Her book jacket describes her as having received an A.B. *magna cum laude* from Harvard in 1989, and a Yale Law School degree in 1992. In 1995, she received a M.F.A. from Cornell's graduate writing program. She has clerked for federal appellate and trial judges in Boston and New York, and now lives in Washington, D.C. where she works as a litigator practicing criminal defense and First Amendment law. In between all of this, she managed to write what I believe is the most accurate portrayal of the suffering that Alzheimer's disease can cause for children in dysfunctional caregiving families.

The Bad Daughter painfully recounts Hildon's need to withdraw from her mother's illness and her demanding family. She recalls her initial escape from her demented mother during her first days at Harvard:

I knew I could make myself up there at college, perhaps from books, creating a persona that could be punctured, that was built on paper, but that could also be animated and become real. It struck me that night and then more deeply, that the wall, or perhaps the bridge of books that I'd been building was complete. I believed that I'd successfully left my mother in order to live in books, in the space they created.[6]

Despite Hildon's success in creating her escape, her mother's sister, Aunt Betty, continued to make demands that she assume responsibility for her mother's care. To some readers, the demands may not seem so unreasonable. At several points during the memoir, Hildon's aunt asks her to help by saying that, "It's time for you to do your part. Why don't you come out to Tucson and help me move her into a home, and we can figure out a place for you to work here for a while. Later, we can trade off taking care of your mother. I'll do it for a few years, then you can do it for a few years."[7]

When Hildon did not respond, her aunt increased her demands, and in one telephone conversation insisted: "You come out here Julie, you come out here right now." Hildon stated that she "hung up on her, out of panic." She recalls: "This can't happen. Not now, not after years of school, not when my real life is just about to begin. I had fled so far, . . . so successfully."[8] For Hildon, although her aunt was a devoted and loving caregiver, she recalls that her aunt became a "nightmare" for her because of the persistent demands for help: "There was no middle ground for her. I had to move to Tucson and leave school. Later, I had to accept my several year rotation as the primary person to care for my mother."[9]

For the several-year duration of her mother's illness, Hildon's aunt continually berated her for failing to take responsibility for her mother's care, and constantly reminded her of the many sacrifices that she had made so that Julie could continue to escape from her mother. At one point, Hildon says of her aunt: "She taunted me, crowing that I had Alzheimer's on both sides. She told me that I'd get mine, one way or the other. My just desserts would come to me, she said. She told me I was a bad person."[10]

Like many successful escapees from dysfunctional caregiving families, Hildon realized that she could not become reinvolved in the highly stressed family dynamics, even as her mother was dying from the disease. However, Hildon's attempts to wall herself off from her past opened the door to a life of dysfunctional friendships and a series of unfulfilling love relationships.

This painful but engaging and beautifully written book is a reminder that children are indeed the true victims of Alzheimer's disease. The dysfunctional caregiving family response creates several victims. While Hildon portrays herself throughout her memoir as the bad daughter, those good daughters and sons who become Super-Helpmates to their martyred-caregiving parent also pay a heavy price.

The Super-Helpmate role for children appears at first to be the more acceptable one. Children of Martyr-Caregivers and Super-Caregivers actually learn to become Super-Helpmates by watching the caregiving dynamics in the household. They are far more likely to evolve in compatible families in which there is little conflict and family members appear to agree with one another about most issues. Still, while there is no overt conflict, children in these apparently compatible families may also be suffering because their needs are not being met. The expectations for them are often too high, as children in dysfunctional caregiving families seem to have lost their place as the child in the family, a role which is now assumed by an increasingly demented parent or grandparent. These children are deprived of the attention, love, and affection of at least one parent, since the consumed caregivers channel most of their energy and emotion into the caregiving role.

While these Super-Helpmates continue to perform well in school and graciously help with the caregiving, they too are suffering as much as the escapees described above. They are just suffering in silence. If the caregiving goes on too long, these children are also in danger of desiring to escape from the dysfunctional caregiving family. Some of them will never return.

TOWARD POSITIVE OUTCOMES FOR CAREGIVING CHILDREN

Although there is much evidence that children in many Alzheimer's caregiving families feel a deep sense of frustration resulting from constrained family relationships, recent research has indicated that there are children in Reality-Based households who actually benefit from the caregiving process. Diane Beach's most recent study found that the Alzheimer's eldercare experience resulted in a number of positive relationship-building opportunities for family members.

Some caregiving adolescents found themselves growing closer to the primary caregiver and engaging in more activity time with brothers and sisters. For them, the caregiving facilitated closer family bonds. One adolescent described his relationship with his mother as they both cared for his father, an early-onset Alzheimer's victim: "My mother and I became closer . . . we had to lean on each other for support while I was at home and so we became dependent upon each other."[11]

Another adolescent whose father had Alzheimer's recalls: "Well, my brother used to come down from Fullerton maybe once a month or once every two months. Now he comes down a lot and we go out with my dad. And then on Saturday and Sunday, we'll play racquetball or something like that which we never had done before."[12]

One adolescent grandchild of an Alzheimer's victim stated:

We were out to dinner one night and I was with my grandparents and there were some other family members there too. My grandma asked the same question five times incessantly and did not realize she was doing it. The only way we can really handle it is to just sort of laugh about it and say, oh well that's just the way it is. We give each other looks as if to say, "whatever." In a way, that helps us to be closer and to be able to relieve the tension through kidding each other.

These positive caregiving outcomes are only possible, however, when the family caregiving dynamics create a Reality-Based Caregiving environment that is supportive of each family member's needs. Martyr-Caregiving and Super-Caregiving families will never lend themselves to the development of a positive nurturing family environment in which the needs of all family members are considered.

A Reality-Based Caregiving environment is one in which there are realistic goals, coupled with attention to the needs of all in the family, especially the children. But this is much more difficult to accomplish, because the needs of the Alzheimer's patient seem so overwhelming in comparison with those of a seemingly independent adolescent child. Too often the needs of the child are neglected in favor of attending to the more pressing demands of the Alzheimer's patient. Children and adolescents often grow to resent this.

In response to what is now becoming a serious caregiving concern, the Alzheimer's Association offers a program targeted to children and adolescents in caregiving families. The "Kids Care" Program offers an opportunity for caregiving children and adolescents to meet together in a group for information sharing, open discussion, and social activities. In the groups, children have the opportunity to discuss shared issues and concerns. It is especially helpful for children to learn that their feelings of ambivalence and resentment are often shared by other caregiving children. This mutual validation and support is invaluable for many children.

In addition to the children's support group, the Alzheimer's Association has books and films for children which are available for rent. For example, a film entitled *Just for the Summer* was perfect for us because its main character is a boy just about Jonathan's age. The film describes the family dynamics which evolve as the boy's Alzheimers-impaired grandmother moves in with the family "just for the summer." This offered an excellent opportunity for our family to talk about how our experiences were similar to those of the family in the film. Although Jonathan said that the grandmother in the film was "nowhere near as bad as Nana," viewing the film together gave us an opportunity to talk about our concerns.

Looking back on our three caregiving years, I cannot honestly say that there were positive outcomes for Jonathan, especially during the first year. Despite the increased time spent with his father, it was not until the caregiving demands lessened during the second and third caregiving years that Jonathan once again began to feel his needs were as important as Katharine's.

What could we have done differently? I have learned from our mistakes, and those of many other family caregivers I have met, that the most important thing a caregiving family has to learn is the need for respite care. The family must have time away from the impaired loved one. At the beginning, we tended to try to include Katharine in our family outings and dinner table conversations. We felt guilty if we did not take

Katharine to church or out to dinner with us. However, when Jonathan began refusing to accompany us on some of these outings, we became increasingly concerned and finally began to reconsider our priorities.

Families need to acknowledge that although the impaired family member may have the loudest and seemingly most immediate demands for attention, there are often children in the very same home whose silent needs are being ignored. I have learned that some of the loneliest children are those who live in an Alzheimer's household.

NOTES

1. Elaine Brody, *Women in the Middle: The Parent Care Years* (New York: Springer, 1990).

2. Diane Beach, "Family Care of Alzheimer's Victims," *The American Journal of Alzheimer's Care and Related Disorders and Research* (January/February 1994): p. 15.

3. Beach, "Family Care of Alzheimer's Victims," p. 15.

4. Beach, "Family Care of Alzheimer's Victims," p. 16.

5. Beach, "Family Care of Alzheimer's Victims," p. 16.

6. Julie Hildon, *The Bad Daughter* (Chapel Hill, NC: Algonquin Books, 1988), p. 28.

7. Hildon, *The Bad Daughter*, p. 44.

8. Hildon, *The Bad Daughter*, p. 44.

9. Hildon, *The Bad Daughter*, p. 45.

10. Hildon, *The Bad Daughter*, p. 46.

11. Beach, "Family Care of Alzheimer's Victims," p. 14.

12. Beach, "Family Care of Alzheimer's Victims," p. 14.

Chapter 5

❈

Solutions for the Reluctant Caregivers

It is not easy for caregiving family members to admit that they can no longer provide care without help. This is especially true for Super-Caregivers or Martyr-Caregivers, whose egos are strongly invested in the success of the caregiving. Eventually, they realize, as we did, that caring for an Alzheimer's patient is much too difficult to try to continue alone.

After a long summer without a break from caregiving and a growing decline in our family life, we finally came to the realization that we too needed help. Our initial choice had been to try to manage the caregiving by hiring live-in help. We believed that a full-time paid caregiver would give us the respite we needed, and it did occasionally allow us some free time. However, the demands of an active Alzheimer's patient like Katharine were far too burdensome for one person to handle. While most of the time Katharine was calm and easygoing, we found that she would become difficult and easily upset if any kind of demands were placed on her, including showering, dressing, and going to bed. We learned not to make demands, and allowed her to do whatever she wanted to do. The only problem with that strategy was that it placed extra burdens on the caregiver. We lost several paid caregivers who quickly learned that full-time caregiving for Katharine was one of the most demanding jobs they ever had.

In an attempt to decrease the burden of the caregiving, but still be-lieving that we needed to continue to manage the care at home, we tried hiring shift workers, assuming that if the caregiving was shared by several aides, Katharine could not possibly wear them all out. We found, however, that the lack of continuity made Katharine more confused than ever, and she often became oppositional and even combative with several of the caregiving aides.

Worse, the constant staff turnover also created an unending job for us in orienting each worker to Katharine's needs, demands, and special routines. I had learned much earlier that if Katharine were not ap-proached in a quiet, easygoing manner, she would have what many Alz-heimer's patients experience—a "catastrophic reaction." This is an out-of-control response, much like a child's tantrum. Katharine never had these reactions with us as caregivers, because we had learned how to deal with her. Katharine could never be pushed or forced to take a shower, eat her breakfast, or get dressed. We learned that flexibility, a sense of humor, and a relaxed nature worked best with Katharine, as it does with all Alzheimer's patients. If she wanted to wait to eat breakfast until "her mother arrived," it was fine with us. She would eat eventually.

However, many of the well-intentioned aides felt that Katharine needed to shower and dress according to their schedules. We all paid a heavy price for their rigidity. Over the course of the next few months, Katharine had several catastrophic reactions, often throwing bowls of cereal or plates of eggs at well-meaning caregivers who simply did not understand how to deal with a severely cognitively impaired patient. Not surprisingly, Katharine was not a favorite placement for many of the agency-based aides we attempted to hire. I imagined that there was a picture of Katharine somewhere on the wall of each home health care agency with a warning beneath it. Most caregiving agencies allow their aides to request their placements, and Katharine's care was not a desir-able choice. While we were eventually able to find some excellent aides to cover the day shift, evenings and nights were left for us to manage by ourselves. Stress levels were at an all-time high for all of us, because school was back in session and we were busy night and day. We were truly at a loss about what to do; we knew we could not continue this level of caregiving for much longer.

We tried to find options. I had earlier considered day-care programs for Katharine, but had dismissed this option because I believed that Katharine was far too advanced in her disease to be accepted for place-ment. At the UCSD evaluation, we learned that she would not qualify for the Alzheimer's Association "Morning Out" day-care program. We finally began to talk seriously about finding a placement outside our home for Katharine.

FINDING A PLACEMENT

While it took us several months to admit that we could not possibly continue the level of care we were providing to Katharine in our home, we had no idea that even after we were ready to place Katharine, we were just beginning another long and frustrating journey. In many ways, our search for an appropriate placement for Katharine became even more frustrating than her actual caregiving had been. We learned that nursing homes do not exactly welcome patients like Katharine. In our search for a home for her, we joined the countless other families of Alzheimer's victims who struggle to find institutional care for their loved ones. Today, I would advise any family whose loved one is diagnosed with Alzheimer's disease to begin the process of choosing a placement as soon as possible. Because we had been so confident that we had the financial resources and caregiving expertise to provide care for Katharine at home, we never even considered looking at outside placements. We were later sorry for this arrogance.

We now know that choosing a facility takes a great deal of time and energy. Nearly all good nursing homes have long waiting lists, and more importantly, not all nursing homes will welcome an Alzheimer's-impaired patient.[1] In theory, a nursing home cannot decline admission to a patient with Alzheimer's disease if the patient meets the eligibility requirements. In practice, many homes turn away these patients by stating that there is no bed available, even if there is one.

To address this problem, caregiving families should never ask on the telephone if the home accepts patients with Alzheimer's disease. Instead, I would suggest to simply ask whether there are available beds. In reality, after phone calls and visits to more than twenty nursing homes throughout San Diego, I was rarely able to receive an answer to the simple question of whether a bed was available. The response was always the same: they would have to "determine the level of care that the patient needed." I believe now that this was code for "we need to see how much trouble this patient will cause for us before we decide to accept her." Not surprisingly, many families of Alzheimer's patients have a very hard time finding placements for their impaired loved ones.

After a while, we convinced ourselves that we would not have wanted the type of nursing home that was unwilling to accept a patient like Katharine. We assumed that these homes probably did not have adequately trained staff who were familiar with the special behavioral demands of dementia patients. Our negative experience with a number of poorly trained caregiving aides taught us that it takes a very special person with specialized training to know how to respond to an Alzheimer's patient. We were looking for caregiving personnel whose knowledge, abilities, and personalities would enable them to provide loving, patient, and supportive care. We became discouraged.

Finally, with help from the Southern Caregivers Alliance, a San Diego-based referral service, we began to look more closely at some of San Diego's "board and care" facilities. We learned that these facilities often had special units for ambulatory Alzheimer's patients. Although these homes are not skilled nursing facilities, most offer secure custodial care. Most of those with the Alzheimer's units have trained caregiving aides who assist residents with personal care, including bathing, dressing, and assistance with eating. Many of the units have social activities for the residents which are geared to the unique needs of the demented population they serve.

ALZHEIMER'S FACILITIES

There are usually two major requirements for admission to these specialized Alzheimer's facilities: First, the patient must be mobile; he or she may use a walker, but cannot be confined to a chair or bed. Second, the behavior of the Alzheimer's patient must be manageable, so that they will not present a risk to the other residents. These are typical requirements for most state-approved board and care Alzheimer's facilities.

We knew that Katharine certainly met the mobility requirement. Actually, it was her constant mobility that presented the most problems to her caregivers. However, we were concerned about the second requirement. While we never had problems with Katharine's behavior, we knew that untrained caregiving aides did. But, we assumed that the staff in an Alzheimer's facility would be able to deal with the behavioral challenges she might present. With renewed hope, we began to turn our attention to the board and care Alzheimer's facilities in San Diego county.

Each weekend, my husband and I would visit one or two of the facilities to try to determine whether they might be appropriate for Katharine. At the beginning of our search, we were both seriously distressed by our initial visits to the Alzheimer's units. This was our first real exposure to the sights and sounds of large numbers of demented elderly people. While many of the residents seemed to be engaged in activities in some of the units, others were gesturing at imaginary things in the air or talking incoherently to invisible people; one resident was picking the "flowers" off of the wallpaper. It was especially disturbing for Dana to see these facilities. We both had to admit, however, that many of the residents looked and acted a lot like Katharine.

One facility was particularly disconcerting for us. When we drove up to this facility, we noticed that behind its large gates and fences, six or seven of the elderly residents were walking alone and quite purposefully on a path that encircled the facility. The path had become so warn down that it actually had become like a jogging track. I learned later that this track was one of the ways that the facility was able to accommodate the "wanderers." As we watched, each of the walkers on that path had a determined look on their faces, as if they knew exactly where they were going and that they needed to get to an important appointment or event. There was no conversation among the walkers, as each walked alone, each with a specific goal. We could only imagine what that goal might have been. For Katharine, we know it would have been her childhood home from long ago. In our San Diego home, Katharine would prepare to leave each evening after dinner to go back "up home" to the farm because she said her mother and brothers were waiting for her there. We guessed that perhaps school or work awaited the determined walkers. We realized that to call them wanderers is incorrect, because the word "wander" connotes a moving around without a definite purpose or objective. Alzheimer's patients always have a purpose—their determined steps, the firm jaws, and the eyes straight ahead all dispute the word "wander."

Whatever the personal goal of each of the walkers, it was rather worrisome for us to see this busy walking, considering the fact that the temperatures in the early fall of East County San Diego regularly rise higher than ninety degrees. It seemed dangerous to us, although we later learned that many of these Alzheimer's facilities, try to leave the main residence unlocked so that the residents can feel they have ultimate freedom to go outside. There were no restraints used, or locked units, and this feature was viewed as a "plus" when evaluating Alzheimer's facilities. We found that many of these special facilities had large fences which encircled the grounds to safely enclose the wanderers, who would most likely spend hours going in circles around the facility. This "freedom" was one of many creative ways these facilities tried to address the problematic pacing or wandering behavior so characteristic of Alzheimer's patients.

Still, touring the facilities was difficult for us. Invariably, at least one or two of the residents would ask us to please call their mother for them. Often, residents would try to follow us out the locked gates toward our car as we would leave. We often had to stay inside, waiting at the gate until a staff member arrived to distract the potential escapee long enough to allow us to exit the gates.

These visits were discouraging, and we had real reservations about even considering any of these units as a placement for Katharine. Yet, we had to admit that she would have fit right in with these demented residents. After two months of visiting these facilities, we agreed on a possible placement for her.

The facility we chose was in bucolic East County San Diego, about a thirty-minute drive from our home. Surrounded by hills and beautiful trees, we thought Katharine would be reminded of her childhood farm home. The thirty-bed facility was entirely devoted to Alzheimer's patients, and therefore had many programs and activities designed for their special needs. Katharine had passed the intake interview easily. The director of the facility was especially impressed by Katharine's remarkable energy levels and walking ability. While extremely confused, Katharine was her most gracious, cooperative, and talkative self. When the administrator asked Katharine if she would like to stay at the facility, she responded that she would like to stay, but advised the director that she would have to check with her mother first.

We allowed ourselves to hope that Katharine might possibly be out of our home and into a safe, secure, and loving environment by Christmas. The paperwork took little time, and since we were a "full-private pay" family, there was no need for applications for financial assistance. It was decided that Katharine would move to the facility in mid-December.

The next few weeks were spent preparing for her move. As if she was going to camp, I sewed name tags into all of Katharine's clothing, as well as her blankets and pillowcases. We purchased a supply of her favorite toiletries, and packed some family pictures to place on her nightstand. Everything seemed easier at home, because we finally knew that there was an end in sight. At this point, we were certainly ready to let go of our home-based caregiving.

On the other hand, Katharine of course had no recollection that she had even visited the facility, but since she had so enjoyed the interview process, I was confident that the well-trained staff would help her make a good adjustment. Once again, however, I seriously underestimated

Katharine's behavior and overestimated the abilities of the caregiving staff at this facility.

ANOTHER DISAPPOINTMENT

We arrived at the facility shortly before lunchtime on a sunny December morning. The welcoming staff fussed over Katharine, and brought us to her lovely private room which overlooked the East County hills. She had a sliding glass door to the secured "outside" and could therefore join the other walkers in their daily perimeter walks whenever she chose. I began to unpack Katharine's clothing and arranged her locked closet. As Katharine sat on the bed in her new room, I placed family photographs on the dresser and put her toothbrush in the bathroom. She seemed happy, and mentioned several times how pretty the trees outside her room were.

As I was completing the unpacking, one of the friendly aides invited Katharine to join the other residents for lunch in the dining room. The kind aide offered to take Katharine to the dining room and said I could join them when I had finished the unpacking. After about ten minutes, the facility director came rushing back to me. She looked frightened, and I worried that Katharine had fallen. Instead, she told me that Katharine was "acting out," which I now know is code for "having a major tantrum," and would have to leave. As I rushed back to the dining room, I thought she meant that Katharine would have to leave the dining room. She didn't. She meant that Katharine would have to leave the facility.

Apparently, in the ten minutes that Katharine was away from me in the unfamiliar dining room setting, she had obviously become terrified and responded with violence. It could have been something so minor as someone asking Katharine what she wanted to eat, or someone else asking her to sit down. Whatever the cause, I learned later that Katharine had overturned several food trays and had attempted to kick the aides who tried to subdue her. Katharine had frightened even these capable and experienced caregivers. There was no way that this East County facility was going to keep her.

I hurriedly packed up her clothes, took the family photographs off the dressers, and in my haste had overstuffed one of the paper shopping bags. As we were unceremoniously exiting the facility, my overloaded Nordstrom's shopping bag broke, and all of Katharine's family photographs and toiletries spilled onto the floor near the front gate. All Katharine could say was, "You do too much shopping." During the ride home, I kept wondering how I would tell Jonathan that nothing had changed, and that we would have to endure this for a while longer. I worried about how I might keep my own sanity as the caregiving became more and more difficult. On a rational level, I could not be angry with Katharine for her behavior at the facility—once we drove away, she had already forgotten that she had ever visited the unit.

But during the drive home, I found myself wishing she were dead. And then I began to worry that I might kill her. These feelings are frightening, and they concern me even today. Wishing someone would die, especially a helpless relative, is very frightening. But I knew how disappointed the rest of the family would be. We had already begun to plan our lives without Katharine, and anticipated a Christmas without the sleepless nights of caregiving. After our East County experience, I began to seriously doubt whether we would ever have our lives back again. But on the long ride home, I finally made the decision to either find a way to get Katharine out of our home, or drastically change our ways of dealing with her. I knew we needed professional help.

FINALLY, FINDING HELP IN THE COMMUNITY

Today, as we look back, the East County experience was in many ways a defining experience for us. We began to discard the Super-Caregiving and Martyr-Caregiving roles, and became even more determined to reclaim our family life. We also knew that our options were limited. We briefly even considered placement in a private psychiatric hospital, which turned out to be the only facility that would accept Katharine. When a person with a dementing illness exhibits behaviors that are so difficult to manage that no nursing home or board and care Alzheimer's facility will accept him or her, psychiatric hospitalization is the only option. But because these facilities were frightening even for us, we delayed consideration until we had tried other options.

We immediately made an appointment for Katharine to return to the UCSD psychiatrist who had been part of her initial evaluation team. With this understanding physician, we began to seriously consider the benefits of medication. Medication was an option that we had rejected in our earlier quest for Super-Caregiving. As a sociologist, I had always dismissed the use of medication as a lazy way to try and manage problematic behaviors. However, at this point, as desperate caregivers, we were ready to try anything.

Sensing our stress and considering Katharine's reactions to the attempted placement, her psychiatrist agreed that we could no longer provide the twenty-four-hour-a-day behavior management that Katharine required. When we fully described and documented Katharine's symptoms and outbursts, she immediately realized that her worsening symptoms required an anti-psychotic drug. She prescribed Risperadone. And, to address Katharine's agitated evening behaviors, she prescribed Trazodone for its antidepressant and sleep-promoting actions. Trazodone was at once effective in improving Katharine's agitation and mood, even with the continued rotation of agency-based caregiving aides. We began to feel hopeful.

Still, the best advice that Katharine's wonderful psychiatrist gave us was to enroll her, as soon as she was stabilized on her medication, in San Diego's Glenner Alzheimer's Family Day Care Center. Glenner was unique, because it was the only day-care center that would indeed be willing to work with even severely demented Alzheimer's patients. The psychiatrist believed that once Katharine was maintained on a low dosage of Risperadone, she would be appropriate for inclusion in the program, and if we desired, we could probably make reapplication to the Alzheimer's facilities that had formerly rejected her. The psychiatrist made the referral to day-care for us, and the center's director called us to invite Katharine for a visit. It was certainly a welcome call for us.

We learned from Katharine's psychiatrist that the personnel at Glenner had all received at least six weeks of full-time course work and training in dementia care. In fact, the center has its own educational program for nurse's aides throughout San Diego County to gain certification in dementia care. We have learned that Glenner provides the most extensive dementia caregiving training to caregivers in California. We began to feel hopeful that if anyone could handle Katharine, it would be the extremely well-trained staff at Glenner. Finally, we were correct in our assumptions!

From the first day that Katharine arrived at the center, there was never a question of whether they could handle her behavior. They loved Katharine, and she loved them. We were so grateful to the workers at the Glenner Center; they soon became our lifeline back to becoming a normal family. Katharine attended the Glenner Center six days each week. While she remembered little of the day's activities, the good feelings she returned home with each day stayed with her through the evening.

Key to the center's success was its full day of constant activities and structure. Each morning, Katharine began her day in the center by participating in the staff-led "current events" discussions. By 10 A.M., Katharine progressed to crafts activities, sing-alongs, bingo (with a lot of help), dancing, supervised walks in the neighborhood, cookie making, and cupcake decorating. In the middle of the day, a hot lunch was provided, and then another walk outdoors accompanied by staff members and two or three other participants. There was not a minute during the day that Katharine was not thoroughly occupied. And she loved every minute of every day at the center.

The nurturing and well-trained workers never made demands upon the participants, except to ensure their safety. They understood that Alzheimer's victims can never be forced to do things. They chose to allow the patients to see how much fun they would miss if they did not join in. And, in response, most of the participants happily joined all of the activities because the staff was just so enthusiastic and fun-loving. I have never met such an energetic group of caregivers! They are "up" and involved at all times. Their enthusiasm is most contagious and all of the participants "caught" onto the fun. Even family members often felt compelled to join the sing-alongs when they arrived to pick up their loved ones at the end of the day. I found myself participating in more than one "tea dance" in the late afternoon!

At the beginning, I wondered how the day-care staff always seemed so happy and engaged with their charges. They stood in sharp contrast to the overworked and exhausted-looking aides I had met at many of the nursing homes and Alzheimer's facilities I had visited. I wondered how they managed to stay so enthusiastic about their work. Later, I found that Glenner has excellent staff-patient ratios, and even more importantly, staff members are encouraged to take frequent breaks during the day. They take what I would call a "tag-team" approach to caregiving, meaning that as one staff member becomes weary, another staff member takes over, having rested sufficiently to take on the work. The Glenner philosophy acknowledges that caregivers must also take care of themselves.

However, I believe this is only part of the explanation for the Glenner success, which has much more to do both with the selection process for caregivers, and to the training they receive. Applicants are screened carefully, and only those with the special enthusiasm and energy for working with Alzheimer's patients are invited to participate in the training. The extensive training that the center director provides to all of the workers is also key to the success, because even enthusiastic caregivers can quickly burn out if they do not understand how to deal with the everyday demands of a severely demented population.

Katharine's days were now full. In addition to the regularly scheduled activities, there were often "special" visitors to Glenner, including wonderful volunteers from the community who arrived each afternoon to entertain the day-care participants. A frequent visitor was an elderly gentleman whose two pet poodles performed "amazing" tricks. Additional visitors included local singers and dancers from area schools, and brownie and girl scout troops who arrived to help Katharine and the others make valentines or Christmas cards. I have kept many of the valentines that Katharine and her "helpers" made for me.

Each morning, as I pulled into the center's driveway, Katharine could hardly wait to get out of the car. Amazingly, she recognized the building each morning. This was surprising, because by this point she hardly recognized the members of her own family. By the third month of her involvement in center activities, she no longer needed the Risperadone. The staff advised that we contact her psychiatrist to see if the dosage could be reduced. They worried that Katharine was becoming too tired to participate in the afternoon walk and sing-alongs. We still maintained her on a low dose of the Trazodone in the evenings so that she (and we) could sleep uninterruptedly.

For the first time in nearly a year, Katharine was happy, We were happy because our house was finally becoming ours. Katharine was out of the house each day from 9 A.M. until 5 P.M. Even when she arrived back home after her wonderfully full day, she was tired and continued to be happy throughout the evening. For the first time since she had moved into our home, she began sleeping through the night, and we all began to feel rested. We stopped looking for a residential placement for Katharine. After the year of a caregiving nightmare, we finally found a solution that worked for all of us, including Katharine.

Life was finally manageable. We still had minor challenges, including occasional scheduling difficulties in transporting Katharine to and from the day-care center. As a dual-career couple, our work demands often interfered with Katharine's scheduled arrival and departure times. Many dual-career couples would probably have had a hard time trying to combine work and caregiving if they depended upon the 9 A.M. opening for day care. I was fortunate to have a family-friendly job like university teaching. I was able to design my teaching schedule around the opening and closing of the center, just as I had done for our children. Still, as the following chapter demonstrates, there are increasing numbers of families who are now trying to juggle work schedules with caregiving schedules. And many of these families are trying to accomplish the caregiving without the workplace flexibility we enjoyed.

NOTE

1. Ellen Graham, "A Daughter's Odyssey, A Home for Dad," *Wall Street Journal* (November 11, 1998): pp. 1B, 10B.

Chapter 6

————————————— ❊ —————————————

Family Caregiving and
the Workplace

The Family and Work Institute's most recent "National Study of the Changing Workforce" showed a startling 42 percent of employees expect to assume elder care duties within the next five years. As a dual-career couple, my husband and I joined the many caregivers who are attempting to balance elder caregiving with career commitments. However, unlike most caregivers, our balancing was greatly eased because I had the luxury of a supportive workplace. I was able to draw upon the "family-friendly flexibility" that university teaching affords, and arrange my teaching and student-advising schedule to coincide with the hours that Katharine attended day care.

Many caregivers do not have this luxury. These workers and their employers are often paying a heavy price. Studies of the impact of the dual roles of elder caregiving and employment have shown that the negative effects of the caregiving are experienced not only by the individual caregiver in terms of stress and physical exhaustion, but also by the workplace itself. The latest research demonstrates that there can be serious workplace consequences when workers must attend to the care of an elderly loved one. According to information from a survey compiled by Work-Family Directions, a Boston consulting firm, findings indicated that employees caring for an elderly relative miss an average of five workdays each year.[1] Even when these caregiving employees are at work, they often experience a number of difficulties, including distracting phone calls, loss of vacation time, stress from trying to catch up on work due to unexpected time off, tardiness, and early departures from work.

An estimate of the expense to the employer was offered in the business periodical *INC* as about $2,500 per year, per employee, in lost productivity due to elder caregiving. [2] There is growing evidence that this estimate is too low.[3]

WORKPLACE COSTS OF ELDER CAREGIVING

Several factors contribute to the hidden costs that employers already bear for elder care. A recent study for Metropolitan Life Insurance found that each year, at least 5 percent of all caregiving employees quit their jobs altogether to care for an older parent. An estimated 11 percent of all caregivers take off an average of six days a year to provide routine care, while more than half of all caregivers average three days a year dealing with elder-care crises. Other costs include the extra managerial time needed to supervise and cover for caregivers who need to take time off, as well as the high demand placed by some caregivers on health insurance benefits and mental health services.

Stressed caregivers' late arrivals, long lunch breaks, and early departures also take a toll on the workplace, as missed time negatively affects productivity. Other workers may begin to resent covering for the missing caregiver, and this creates disharmony in the workplace. These disruptions are not nearly as problematic as the workday interruptions faced by caregivers who need to spend work time talking on the phone with anxious loved ones, or the lost work hours spent by the caregiver who spends work time on the phone making arrangements with service providers. This situation can arise even for the employees who do not physically care for parents, or for those whose parents live elsewhere. Estimated at one hour per week per caregiver, this factor is the biggest drain of all on employee productivity, amounting to well over half of the estimated total cost for employee caregiving.

In addition to declines in worker productivity due to family caregiving, there are often issues of worker attitude, which can negatively affect the bottom line of many companies. For example, Donna Klein, director of Marriott International's work-life programs, stated in *American Demographics* that since Marriott's business success depends on excellent customer service, the mood of its employees is extremely important. A worker who is anxious about elder caregiving may not be the most patient and helpful customer service representative. Although the average Marriott worker is just 35 years old, 15 percent of Marriott's workers indicate that they have elder-care responsibilities. In companies with an older worker population, that number is much higher.[4]

A survey of one thousand American workers conducted by Hilton Hotels Corporation found that for many of their employees, the years from age thirty to fifty are often "lost" to meeting the needs of other people, including children and aging parents. According to John Robinson, director of the University of Maryland's Americans' Use of Time Project, "It is clear that Americans in this group face enormous family-career conflicts."[5] The findings about the particular struggles of the thirty to fifty age group were so definitive that the study authors referred to that stage of life as the "lost years."

For caregivers of Alzheimer's patients, the demands and extended length of the caregiving commitment create serious conflicts for those who are trying to combine caregiving with a career. These workers often begin to feel hopeless, and may leave the workplace. Companies are paying the price for these "lost employees," and some of them are beginning to respond to these losses. Still, the first task of employers is to determine exactly how great the problem is, and this is much easier said than done.

THE PREVALENCE OF WORK-FAMILY CAREGIVING CONFLICTS

Determining exactly how many employees are struggling, or are expected to struggle with elder caregiving is much more complex than it first appears. Still, it is important to try to estimate the number of employees who are currently or are expected to assume elder caregiving roles, so that those in the workplace can be prepared. A lack of information of the prevalence and the impact of elder caregiving by employees has caused many companies to be reluctant to respond to caregiving concerns. Many companies simply do not even know the extent of the elder care problems that their employees are facing. Sociologists and gerontologists have not been especially helpful either, because the previous research on the prevalence of elder caregiving by employees failed to address the complexity of the issue.

If we look simply at the rate of employment in samples of caregivers drawn from national and regional studies, these caregivers' studies consistently report that approximately 40 percent of all caregivers are employed. Yet, when we look at studies by corporations themselves, we have much more inconsistency with elder caregiving prevalence rates,

ranging from a low of 2 percent[6] of all employees in a major manufacturing plant study of caregiving, to more than 35 percent for large corporations which employ large numbers of women.[7] Such
inconsistencies in assessing the prevalence of elder caregiving is confus-
ing at best, and has been of little use to employers in determining the
costs of elder caregiving for their companies.[8]

A study by Metropolitan Life Insurance Company attempted to
quantify more precisely the impact of elder-care costs on employers.
The study applied a model of elder-care costs to a manufacturing firm
with about 87,000 salaried employees and found that the total employer costs were more than $5.5 million each year. And this analysis
probably underestimated the extent of elder care done in most companies, because at this particular manufacturing plant under study, only
about 2 percent of the firm's employees provided actual physical help to
older relatives in the form of assistance with eating, bathing, and dressing.[9]

This 2 percent estimate is most likely low, because the manufacturing
plant under study in the Metropolitan Life Study was a highly male-
skewed workforce. We have already seen that women are significantly
more likely than men to provide elder care, and because of this, organizations with larger shares of female employees can expect much higher
elder care-related costs.

Evidence of this is provided in two recently completed corporate
surveys by the Boston University Center on work and family. Of the
two companies, the company with a 75 percent male workforce had a 4
percent rate of employee elder caregiving, while the company with a 60
percent female workforce found that 13 percent of the employees reported caregiving responsibilities. If we used the 13 percent prevalence
of caregivers in the workforce, we would estimate employer "hidden
costs" for elder care in a plant of 87,000 employees to reach $33 million
per year.[10]

Employers are now beginning to learn that in order to assess caregiving costs, the company size, type of industry, and geographic location
all influence employee caregiving prevalence rates. Many of these or-
ganizational characteristics are also correlated with the demographics
of gender and age composition of the company's workforce. All of
these demographic characteristics will affect caregiving concerns. For
example, a large New England insurance company with high numbers
of female employees is likely to have much higher numbers of family
caregivers in need of support. In contrast, a large West Coast manufacturing company with a highly male-skewed workforce is more likely to

have only about 2–3 percent of their employees balancing work and elder care. As a result, caregiving costs for employers vary greatly, and the response to the caregiving needs of their employees should also vary greatly.

EMPLOYER RESPONSES TO ELDER CAREGIVING CONCERNS

In response to growing employee concerns about family caregiving and its effects upon employee satisfaction and corporate productivity, many firms are taking a proactive approach by offering elder-care assistance to their employees. Increasing corporate interest in helping employees handle their work-family conflicts has resulted in the development of employer-sponsored policies, benefits, and programs. There are many gerontologists and human resource executives who had called workplace–elder-care programs the "benefit of the '90s,"[11] because it seemed that these benefits were quickly becoming a component of the work-family benefit package of many American employers. In the early nineties, there were the beginnings of some highly visible elder-care programs.

IBM, whose nationwide elder-care referral service had received considerable media attention, was described as having been developed as a "proactive response" to undeniable demographic trends.[12] IBM was one of the earliest leaders in responding to the graying of the population that had been predicted by demographers for decades.

This attention to employee elder-care needs has been occurring in Canada for some time now. In 1989, fewer than 6 percent of all Canadian organizations surveyed by the Conference Board of Canada provided an elder-care information and referral service. By 1994, this number had increased to 20 percent.[13] Additional forms of assistance include flexible working hours, work-at-home arrangements, job sharing, and family-related leave. Some companies actually provide financial assistance or subsidies to help staff in covering the costs of providing care to the elderly. These companies recommend cash vouchers for dependent care and subsidized travel for elder-care responsibilities. Canadian businesses have been typically more responsive to the societal demands upon workers' time and energy. At present, 46 percent of Canadian employers are providing some type of elder-care assistance.

While somewhat slower to respond to these elder-care concerns, American companies are now beginning to acknowledge the difficulties faced by many employees who are providing assistance to elderly relatives. A few years ago, twenty-one United States corporations jointly launched a $25.4 million initiative to develop dependent-care projects in communities across the country. Corporate leaders from IBM, AT&T, Aetna Life and Casualty, Exxon, Xerox, Chevron Corporation, and others joined forces to directly address work-family issues, including elder caregiving and child care. What is called the American Business Collaboration for Quality Dependent Care is now credited with enlisting more than 156 businesses, government entities, and not-for-profit organizations to invest more than $27 million in forty-five communities located in twenty-five states.[14] While many of these programs are devoted to providing child care, some of the elder-care initiatives include consultation services, reimbursement accounts, intergenerational day-care centers, and emergency financial assistance for caregiving emergencies. In 1997, this collaboration entered a second phase, with a $100 million initiative to further its mission over the next six years.

AT&T's Family Care Development Fund helps employees to create community-based solutions to their dependent-care problems. AT&T, along with the Communications Workers of America and the International Brotherhood of Electrical Workers of America, invested $25 million in 1,700 programs for child care and elder care throughout the country.[15] The fund addresses employee needs by providing information and support, offering financial assistance (including reimbursement accounts that allow employees to set aside money in pretax dollars for elder-care expenses), and flexible work arrangements. The fund also improved local community services and adult day-care services. In addition, AT&T facilitates focus groups to assess caregivers' needs in various locations throughout the country, offers caregiver support groups in ten cities, and sponsors elder-care fairs. The commitment that AT&T has made to assisting employees with elder care is extraordinary. This may be due, in part, to the larger-than-average need for elder-care assistance for the female-skewed employee population of AT&T. Other companies typically offer far less assistance.

At present, the most prevalent assistance program included dependent-care spending accounts for elder-care, and unpaid leaves of absence. Companies are also beginning to offer elder-care referral sources. Each of these programs has advantages and disadvantages, but researchers are finding that despite what seems to be the good faith efforts of many employers, employees continue to be reluctant to draw upon these elder-care benefits.

EMPLOYEE RELUCTANCE TO USE
EMPLOYER-SUPPORTED ELDER-CARE SUPPORT

Many corporate leaders are not convinced that work-family issues like elder-care are a business concern, or that these policies will have a positive effect on worker productivity. And low worker usage of these programs seems to indicate that these corporate leaders may indeed be correct. This, coupled with the long battle over a national family and medical leave policy, reflects the nature of the business community's reluctance to adopt family-oriented benefits. The passage of the Family and Medical Leave Act of 1993 requires employers with fifty or more employees to grant up to twelve weeks of unpaid leave annually when a child is born or adopted, or when an immediate family member with a serious health condition needs care. Leave is also granted when the employee is unable to work because of a serious health condition. Employers must maintain any preexisting health coverage during the leave period, and once the leave is completed, reinstate the employee to the same or an equivalent job.

While employers were concerned about the potential burden of maintaining the health insurance coverage for employees on leave and the expenses of recruiting and training replacement workers, the reality is that few workers take advantage of these leaves of absence. When they are used, women are more likely to use these leaves than men, and they are seldom used for elder care.

The protracted nature of Alzheimer's caregiving makes it impossible to predict the length of time needed for caregiving. Twelve weeks would certainly be insufficient. As importantly, however, most employees cannot afford to give up their salary for up to twelve weeks. While higher-paid managers and professionals may be able to afford the financial loss more easily than the line workers, the social stigma of lower career expectations for those taking these leaves is significant. Upwardly mobile employees have learned that elder caregivers may be viewed as having a divided commitment to work and family. And, even in today's apparent support for work-family issues, those who do not demonstrate total commitment to the workplace are viewed negatively when promotions, raises, and bonuses are being considered.

In contrast, dependent-care accounts are often part of an overall flexible benefits plan, and are allowed under Internal Revenue Code provisions stating that employer payments for dependent-care expenses may be excluded from an employee's annual taxable income. By placing deductions from an employee's paycheck into a reimbursement account, the employee is able to use pretax dollars for dependent-care expenses. The employer incurs no additional costs other than administrative.

Although many companies currently provide dependent-care accounts as an option to employees, most firms report relatively low usage. One researcher attributes this to the fact that salary reduction plans are most useful to the small group of higher-income employees. Most employees are reluctant to enlist programs which will reduce the amount of their paycheck, even when the tax savings are significant. A second reason that employees are not using the reimbursement accounts is because of the complexity of federal regulations governing these accounts. Regulations create difficulties for employees, because they are required to predict their care expenses one year in advance. Anticipating elder caregiving expenses one year in advance is almost impossible, since there are so many unanticipated expenses associated with elder care in general, and Alzheimer's care in particular. For those families who use day-care services, the dependent-care accounts can provide significant tax savings, especially for the higher-income family. But this reimbursement account option, like the leave of absence option, emphasizes the controversial aspects of these programs, in that equal access to these benefits may depend entirely upon an employee's economic conditions. Both favor employees with incomes in the higher tax brackets. Both options offer little to employees most in need of assistance. As a result, low usage of employer-provided elder-care assistance continues.

The reality remains that employer-provided elder-care assistance has done little to address issues of work–elder-care conflicts, and the employers who have attempted to offer dependent-care services to employees with elder-care concerns have found that the service itself can be divisive in the workplace.

EMPLOYEE RESISTANCE

A recent study reported in *Public Personnel Management* found that employer support for elder care can actually divide employees. The authors suggest that "strong emotions prevail on both sides of the issue with individuals in need of assistance demanding employer support on one side, and employees without need, demanding equitable distribution of benefit funds on the other."[16] Employees with elder caregiving or child-care needs in the past may additionally feel disgruntled that the company is now helping others, when they themselves had to manage without help.

Employee divisiveness over the desirability of elder-care assistance may have made employers uncertain about whether they too should bring a potentially divisive issue to their companies. This uncertainty, coupled with the growing concern over whether employees will actually use the elder-care services if they are offered, has caused many employers to reconsider the usefulness of these programs.

Conversations with dual-career caregiving families point to what I believe is the major reason that employees are not likely to use the services. It is also the same reason that I would never have considered using employer-provided elder-care assistance. Employees are reluctant to disclose their caregiving commitments. For us, and for many caregiving employees, caring for an elderly family member is a family issue, and not something to bring into the workplace. In addition to these privacy issues, this reluctance to bring caregiving concerns to work comes primarily from employee concerns that they will never again be seen as seriously committed to their careers if they identify themselves as "caregivers." The concern is that when it comes to promotions or raises, they may not be considered because of their elder-care commitments. American corporations continue to value "face time," and those who are more visible at work, and work the longest hours, win the most respect. Caregivers cannot devote as much "face time" to the workplace as others. This is especially true for the upwardy mobile caregiving employees who are most likely to keep their caregiving a secret.

RELUCTANCE TO DISCLOSE CAREGIVING COMMITMENTS

After three years of family caregiving, fewer than five colleagues on my entire campus knew that I was providing in-home care for my Alzheimer's-impaired mother-in-law. With the exception of a very few, trusted friends and colleagues at work, no one knew that before I arrived at work in the morning, I had bathed, dressed, fed, and transported to day care, my elderly mother-in-law. Like the growing number of caregivers who fear that their commitment to their careers might be questioned, I chose to keep my caregiving a secret at work.

The year Katharine moved in with us was the same year that I was being considered for tenure. In universities, this is commonly known as the "critical year," because it is the final year that a faculty member can teach before being awarded tenure. If tenure is denied, the faculty member would no longer be allowed to continue teaching at that university. Fortunately, I had already compiled a long list of publications and funded grant awards. I also had excellent teaching evaluations and a history of strong service to the university and to the community. I had strong peer evaluations, and excellent letters of support from colleagues within the university and throughout the larger academic community. Still, I worried that if my dean or any member of the Promotion and Tenure Committee knew that I was providing extensive caregiving, I too might be denied tenure. For me, these fears were groundless in my supportive Catholic university workplace environment. No faculty member had ever been denied tenure because of child-care or elder-care concerns. Still, there are many universities and other workplace settings where these fears are completely justified.

Professors have been denied tenure at universities for much less reason. For many years, women with young children have been suspected of not being totally committed to their careers. Even today, there are still allegations by female professors who have been denied tenure and believe that they were discriminated against because of their choice to combine parenthood with professor-hood. Most graduate school advisors will suggest that their students delay marriage and childbearing until they are established in their careers. While these concerns are beginning to lessen, many women have such strong worries about untenured childbearing that female professors often wait until they are granted tenure to begin a family. Elder caregiving can be viewed with even more suspicion, because the demands can be even greater than the demands of child rearing. Even after I was awarded tenure and promoted, I did not disclose the caregiving. There are still very few on campus who know that I had ever been the primary caregiver to my mother-in-law.

Caregivers in corporate settings have even more concerns about being viewed as totally committed to their careers. Without the protection of tenure or a strong union, and surrounded by a corporate culture that demands long hours and complete commitment, it would be especially difficult for an upwardly mobile employee to request elder-care benefits to facilitate the caregiving.

In many ways, the discussion about elder-care benefits closely mirrors the contentious response that greeted Harvard Professor Felice Schwartz's 1990 recommendation that businesses provide an alternative track for women who wish to combine family commitments with work responsibilities. Defined by the media as the "Mommy Track," Schwartz suggested that employers should identify and nurture two separate groups. Her suggestion was to treat high-potential "career primary" women, most of whom would be childless, just as if they were talented men. Then, she suggested that companies help career and family women to be productive, but probably not upwardly mobile, by supporting their need for child care and flexible hours. Although Dr. Schwartz, an academic, believed that women could easily move back and forth from one track to the other, the reality of the workplace belies that assertion.[17]

The negative response by feminists to the idea of the "Mommy Track" illustrates the concern that many women continue to feel that once on the "Mommy Track," they will never again be viewed as serious contenders for positions of increasing responsibility. Research shows that they are probably correct. The flexible options available to "family primary" women often create what some researchers call a "velvet coffin" for women—comfortable, but housing a dead career.

A "Caregiver Track" would be even more stigmatizing than the "Mommy Track" for those who chose this option, because of the length of time needed for elder care. It is an unworkable solution for any employee, male or female, who desires to achieve upward mobility in his or her workplace. As the reality of a competitive workplace continues, even in the nonprofit sector, those providing elder care will continue to be reluctant to request assistance from employers with their work-family conflicts. There is still a question for many whether companies should be involved in this family area in the first place, and there are now signs that employers are beginning to find a less stigmatizing and more equitable way to address elder caregiving issues—through the availability of employer-sponsored, long-term health care insurance.

LONG-TERM CARE INSURANCE AS AN AID TO POTENTIAL CAREGIVERS

Earlier this year, the *Wall Street Journal*'s "Work and Family" column proclaimed that "employers are slowly finding their niche in the eldercare picture."[18] The column reported an increase in family-related consultation and planning services. Today, these consultation services go far beyond helping people deal with the "stress" of family demands or simply compiling lists of available nursing homes and day-care services. Today's elder-care services are beginning to include financial and legal planning. More employers are beginning to offer advice and assistance in purchasing employer-sponsored group long-term care insurance for employees and their parents. Employers are finally helping employees plan for the future. Group long-term insurance sign-ups have greatly increased. Employees are beginning to plan for the long term care needs of their parents and themselves. Today, most of these younger employees are not responding to an elder caregiving crisis situation. Instead, they are thoughtfully considering the demographic changes in society and beginning to plan for the future.

One of these younger workers described in The *Wall Street Journal* is Michael Brosler. The *Journal* reports that although Mr. Brosler is only thirty-eight years old, he is already planning ahead for his parents' old age. Though his mother and father are only in their mid-sixties and healthy, Mr. Brosler is urging them to do estate planning. He is also encouraging the idea of long-term care insurance for them. The catalyst for Mr. Brosler and others is watching their parents struggle with caregiving demands of their grand parents. Mr. Brosler has been helping his father care for his grandfather, age ninety-six, now in a $4,000 per month nursing home. Because of this experience, he has learned how complex elder care can be. Like many Americans, Mr. Brosler's family members are living longer, often extending the need for care. The *Journal* reports that Mr. Brosler's great uncle recently died at age 102. He states that "if you want to care for your family, planning ahead for long-term care is one of the best things you can do for them."[19]

The rise in planning is a subtle change in the elder-care/workplace picture. The movement away from trying to provide direct service to caregiving employees is caused by the failure of these earlier employer attempts to meet all of the needs of a growing caregiving population. Most importantly, the access to long-term care insurance through the workplace is an excellent solution to address issues of workplace equity, because all employees can potentially benefit from these policies.

Today's long-term care policies are much better than the "nursing home insurance" of the past. Insurers have learned that people do not want a "nursing home only" policy. Many policies now give equal coverage wherever the impaired person receives it, including in the home, in an adult day-care center, assisted-living facility, or nursing home. The policy should pay if the impaired individual is suffering from Alzheimer's disease or unable to perform any of the activities of daily living, including bathing or dressing.

Some employers are making it easier than ever for employees to access these policies. Lucent Technologies has developed software for long-term planning for employees to use by themselves, so that complete privacy and confidentiality can be maintained. In this way, even employees with immediate concerns about the long-term care of their parents do not have to disclose this information to their employers. Clearly, employers are increasingly comfortable acting as intermediaries for information and insurance. This is a much more appropriate role than a direct-service provider role.

These long-term care policies cannot help those families who are currently providing long-term care to their elderly parents. Understandably, most policies will not cover preexisting conditions like Alzheimer's disease and many other diagnosed illnesses. If employees plan early enough for themselves and their parents by purchasing these policies when they are still healthy and comparatively young, they can prevent the financial devastation that long-term care needs can present. Had we planned early enough, a long-term care policy would have covered Katharine's day-care services and in-home health aides. This policy would have saved our family the more than $100,000 we spent on Katharine's care during the three years we had her in our home. Still, the day-care expenses and health aides enabled us all to continue our commitment to our careers.

THERE'S NO PLACE LIKE WORK

While the double demands of caregiving and work can be overwhelming, many caregivers actually benefit from the workplace distraction. Work becomes a diversion from the stress that Alzheimer's disease caregiving causes. For these workers, the workplace can become a welcome respite. My teaching, research, and university service became an even more important source of self-satisfaction, because the caregiving was so isolating and alienating. As a caregiver, I was as productive at work as I had ever been. I am confident that there were no workplace costs for my employer. In fact, work became a desirable escape, and I was probably even more productive. And once we learned to draw upon the extensive caregiving support network within the day-care system, I was more productive than ever. In fact, without the opportunities for work which brought positive interactions with students, colleagues, and friends, the full-time caregiving role would have been intolerable.

The value of work as respite from caregiving was a consistent theme in my conversations with other caregivers. So often, our common caregiving circumstances encouraged strong friendships among caregivers. I became friends with many of the women who also brought their loved ones to day-care each morning. Many of us were rushing off to jobs throughout the city. One caregiving woman I met as we both struggled to get our loved ones into the center and ourselves to work on time, captured the importance of work in our lives:

Even though getting to work is so hard in the morning, Joe often balks at eating his breakfast or getting dressed. But once I drop him off here, and I am there, I begin to feel sane again. The tension is gone and I drink coffee and talk with people who can carry on intelligent conversations, and I am away from Joe's constant questions. I take calls and handle customer complaints without a stressful thought. By five o'clock I am recharged, because I have had a day of hard work and socializing. I almost begin to miss Joe. I can actually enjoy my evening time with him. I would never quit my job. It keeps me sane.

I felt the same way about the importance of work in my life. Once at work, I had dozens of bright students to teach, and colleagues to share ideas with—so far removed from the isolated reality of home-based caregiving. For me, and for others, work can become a refuge from the relentless demands of caregiving.

To help understand why work has become the haven that the home used to be for most of us, sociologist Arlie Hochschild spent three years studying the changing role of work in the lives of employees of a large corporation. In her book, *The Time Bind*, Hochschild shows how the office is now where employees get to socialize, feel competent, and relax on breaks. Many employees let their workday lengthen for the simple reason that they enjoy it. If home used to be a shelter from the cold, impersonal world of work, for many employees the two have changed places. Now, work is where the heart is—especially for caregivers.

Hochschild sees the phenomenon developing as women flooded into the workforce over the past few decades. Once in a man's world, women readily adopted its values. "Women discovered men's secret," she writes, "They discovered the appeal of work." One of Hochschild's workers said:

I usually come to work early just to get away from the house. I get there at 2:30 P.M and people are there waiting. We sit. We talk. We joke. I let them know what's going on, who has to be where, what changes I have made for the shift that day. We sit there and chitchat for five or ten minutes. There's laughing, joking, fun. My coworkers aren't putting me down for any reason. Everything is done with humor and fun from beginning to end, though it can get stressful when a machine malfunctions.[20]

Of course, this idea of work as a haven is only possible when the care-giver has adequate backup at home or in the community. Work can only be a sanctuary in a heartless world when the workplace itself is a good place to be. I feel fortunate to work in a supportive workplace with sup-portive colleagues.

Certainly, this is not to say that work solves all of the problems of caregiving. This is only to suggest that those caregivers who feel stressed by the double demands of the workplace and the caregiving might want to consider what could become a frightening alternative—a day filled with the often overwhelming and isolated work of caregiving.

NOTES

1. Donna Jenn, "Get Ready for Eldercare," *INC* (September 1995): p. 101.

2. Jenn, "Get Ready for Eldercare," p. 101.

3. Tibbett Speer, "The Unseen Costs of Eldercare," *American Demographics* 18 (June 1996): p. 20.

4. Speer, "The Unseen Costs of Eldercare," p. 21.

5. Wendy Meyers, "Caught in the Middle: Women Caring for Kids and Parents," *Women in Business* 45 (November/December 1993): p. 33.

6. R. Stone and P. Kemper, "Spouses and Children of Disabled Elders: How Large a Consituency for Long Term Care Reform?" *Milbank Quarterly* 67 (1989): pp. 485–506.

7. J. W. Anastas, J. L. Gibeau, and P. J. Larson, "Working Families and Eldercare: A National Perspective in and Aging America," *Social Work* 35 (1990): pp. 405–411.

8. Sharon Tennstedt and Judith Gonyea, "An Agenda for Work and Eldercare Research," *Research on Aging* 16 (1994): pp. 85–109.

9. Speer, "The Unseen Costs of Eldercare," p. 21.

10. Sharon Tennstedt and Judith Gonyea, "An Agenda for Work and Eldercare," p. 88.

11. Donna Wagner and Gail Hunt, "The Use of Workplace Eldercare Programs by Employed Caregivers" *Research on Aging* 19 (1994): pp. 69.

12. Speer, "The Unseen Costs of Eldercare," p. 21.

13. Alexander Mikalachki and Dorothy Mikalachki, "Work-Family Issues: You Had Better Address Them!" *Business Quarterly* 55 (1991): p. 49.

14. Lisa Jenner, "Work-Family Programs: Looking Beyond Written Policies," *Human Resources Focus* 71 (1994): pp. 19.

15. Ellen Galinsky and Peter Stein, "The Impact of Human Resources Polices on Employees," *Journal of Family Issues* 11 (1990): pp. 368–566.

16. Ellen Ernst Kossek and Beverly DeMarr, "Assessing Employees' Emerging Elder Care Needs and Reactions to Dependent Care Benefits," *Public Personnel Management* 22 (1993): p. 617.

17. Felice Schwartz, "Management Women and the New Facts of Life," *Harvard Business Review* (January/February 1989): pp. 65–77.

18. Sue Shellenbarger, "More Children Start Making Plans Early to Care for Elders," *Wall Street Journal* (July 8, 1998): p. 1B.

19. Shellenbarger, "More Children Start Making Plans Early," p. 1B.

20. Arlie Hochschild, *The Time Bind: When Work Becomes Home and Home Becomes Work* (New York: Metropolitan Books, 1997), pp. 37–38.

Chapter 7

❋

Does This Run in the Family?

One of the most frightening aspects of caring for a parent with Alzheimer's is the fear that you too may carry what researchers call the "susceptibility genes" for the disease. It has been recognized for several years that, in many cases, Alzheimer's disease is hereditary—passed down from generation to generation. For caregivers in these families, the caregiving itself can become a terrifying look into the future.

While there has been disagreement among researchers about the inheritability of all types of Alzheimer's, the latest research on familial and hereditary causes of the disease will not provide much reassurance for these caregivers. In fact, a recent book entitled *Candle and Darkness*, by leading Alzheimer's disease researcher, Dr. Joseph Rogers, asserts that "earlier estimates of the inheritability of Alzheimer's disease may have been too low."[1] Until recently, however, researchers had believed that hereditary Alzheimer's disease was relatively rare, and was considered to strike much earlier, at around age 45. In the past, researchers believed that the average age for nonhereditary Alzheimer's was about sixty-five to seventy-five.

Today, it is becoming increasingly clear that these previous estimates may have been too low, with respect to both the age of onset for inherited Alzheimer's disease and also how often inherited Alzheimer's occurs. Now there is evidence that the frequency of genetically determined Alzheimer's disease is much greater than previously thought; in fact, there are scientists who believe that all Alzheimer's disease is inherited.

Still, the inheritability of late-onset Alzheimer's has been more difficult to prove because, as Rogers points out in his book, the hereditary nature of a disease becomes progressively easier to detect when the age of onset is comparatively younger. If a family has an age of onset in the forties or fifties, it is easy to spot the genetic pattern because almost everyone lives long enough to show the symptoms. That may be why scientists previously thought that hereditary Alzheimer's was characterized by an early age of onset; whenever genetic patterns were clear, these patterns were always in relatively young patients. But this does not mean that patients who show the symptoms of Alzheimer's in their seventies or eighties do not also have the inherited form. There simply may not be enough relatives who have lived long enough to show the pattern.

The inheritability issue is one that is often discussed in our family. In my husband's family, there is some anecdotal evidence of a genetic pattern of late-onset Alzheimer's disease, but the evidence we have is not scientific, it is more like the "genetic gossip" that I have noticed characterizes many families with Alzheimer's. This is simply gossip or family talk about patterns of family members who may have died after suffering with what was called in the past, "senility." Although Katharine's own mother died of scarlet fever at age thirty-five without any symptoms of Alzheimer's, both of Katharine's maternal aunts died in their seventies with the senile dementia characteristic of Alzheimer's disease. As was the custom, neither were diagnosed with any disease other than the "senility" of old age.

We continue to ask ourselves whether it was hereditary. It is difficult to say. We would need more information before we could make a judgment on the inheritability of late-onset Alzheimer's disease that seemed to characterize the family, but Katharine's brothers cannot provide this information for us. Two of them died too young to show the symptoms of late-onset Alzheimer's: one brother died in his twenties from tuberculosis, and the other died of heart disease in his mid-fifties. A third brother died in his seventies of heart disease. None showed the symptoms of dementia that Katharine began to exhibit in her seventies. We continue to be uncertain, and wonder whether her brothers might also have developed the disease if they had lived to be as old as Katharine. From the available data about Katharine and her maternal aunts, we might be led to conclude that hereditary Alzheimer's is the verdict. Still, because everyone has already died in Katharine's generation or in earlier generations, there is no data to analyze. We will not know unless future generations begin to show symptoms, or unless members of the next generation decide to have genetic testing done.

Our family is not unique in its uncertainty about its familial and genetic predisposition. Even those who have spent their entire research careers trying to determine the causes of Alzheimer's disease have had great difficulty identifying the genetic patterns for both early- and late-onset Alzheimer's disease. To better understand, it is helpful to first look at some basic facts about genes and the way they work in our lives.

GENES AND ALZHEIMER'S DISEASE

The most comprehensive, yet accessible, explanation of the science of molecular genetics and how this science relates to Alzheimer's disease is the earlier-mentioned *Candle and Darkness*, which is written for the "non-geneticist." Rogers provides us with a thorough understanding of how genetics works in our lives. He first reminds us of what we may have forgotten from our high school science courses. He helps us to recall that our body is built of cells and that every cell within the body is built of molecules. We are then reminded that the instructions for how to build each molecule are contained in the cell's genes. Each gene is like a blueprint for how to build a particular molecule, and the complete set of genes is like a complete set of blueprints for how to build any cell in the body.

Genes occur side by side in long strings called chromosomes. Humans have twenty-three pairs of chromosomes, and an additional pair that determines sex. Within the chromosomes are all of the instructions needed to build all the molecules that make up the cells of the human body. If a small change is made in a gene, a small change is made in the instructions for the molecule that the gene is responsible for. Sometimes even a minor change can be disastrous, as in the cell mutations associated with Alzheimer's disease.[2]

Changes in genes are generally passed on to succeeding generations. Because we know that Alzheimer's disease is hereditary in many families, this is a strong clue that there is a genetic basis for the familial dementia. If there was not a genetic involvement, Alzheimer's could not be handed down from generation to generation.

Several researchers have demonstrated that the connection between Alzheimer's disease and genes has revealed some important findings. One of the most significant outcomes of these investigations has been the discovery of a relationship between Down's syndrome and Alzheimer's. Downs's syndrome is caused by a genetic defect that leads to mental retardation. Instead of having a pair of chromosomes for chromosome 21, Down's victims have what is called "trisomy 21," which means that they have three 21st chromosomes.

How is this related to Alzheimer's disease? In *Candle and Darkness*, Rogers demonstrates that virtually all Down's syndrome patients over the age of thirty-five to forty will show the brain changes that are characteristic of Alzheimer's disease. These Down's patients have the same neuritic plaques throughout the higher brain centers as Alzheimer's patients. Down's patients also have the same neurofibrillary tangles as Alzheimer's patients, and they have the same nerve cell loss. Most importantly, at middle age, the Down's victim is often profoundly demented.[3] For these reasons, Alzheimer's researchers are looking at the genes on chromosome 21 to try and learn more about the disease. Some researchers have already found a gene mutation on chromosome 21 in several families with hereditary Alzheimer's disease patterns.

Although the knowledge about chromosome 21 helps to know how the neuritic plaques are created, this does not help to explain the causes of most cases of hereditary Alzheimer's disease. In fact, only a small percentage of families with hereditary Alzheimer's have a mutation on chromosome 21. There are other gene mutations, including mutations on chromosome 1, which account for a few more families with hereditary Alzheimer's disease.

Still, Rogers asserts that the most promising findings with regard to chromosomal causes of Alzheimer's is the finding of the mutations on chromosome 14. The protein molecule that is built according to the instructions contained in the chromosome 14 gene is called presenilin 1. Mutated changes in presenilin 1 lead to an especially virulent form of Alzheimer's, which strikes earlier than any other gene abnormality. This toxic form of early-onset Alzheimer's has an average age of onset of thirty-five to forty. It is similar to the form described earlier in Julie Hildon's *The Bad Daughter*. In her painful memoir, Hildon writes of the suffering that her mother's early-onset Alzheimer's caused during her teenage and early adult years. Hildon is traumatized by the horrors that the disease brought into her life, and she narrates her concerns about her own genetics as a child of an Alzheimer's victim.

One hypothesis for the cause of this toxic form of early-onset Alzheimer's disease is that the presenilins have something to do with a cellular process called apoptosis. Rogers describes "apoptosis" as a form of "programmed cell death in which, on receipt of the right signals, a cell dutifully commits suicide."[4] This cell death can be adaptive if too many cells are created. However, in Alzheimer's, the apoptosis occurs as an abnormal process. Worse, in the Alzheimer's patient, mutated presenilins do not do their job in opposing apoptosis, and it is allowed to take place when it shouldn't.

While there are severe consequences when these "single-gene" mutations occur, they only explain a small fraction of the total cases of Alzheimer's. Susceptibility genes play a much greater role in predicting most cases of Alzheimer's disease.

THE SUSCEPTIBILITY GENES FOR ALZHEIMER'S DISEASE

Researchers have recently found that although abnormal alterations or mutations of genes can play an important role in hereditary Alzheimer's disease, there is now evidence that genes may play a much more subtle role in hereditary Alzheimer's than is allowed by considering only those which are abnormal or mutated. New research indicates that there may be variants of a particular gene in which one of the variants, though considered normal, can confer increased vulnerability to Alzheimer's disease. This susceptibility gene has turned out to account for many more hereditary cases than the defective genes described earlier.

The first susceptibility gene identified is located on chromosome 19, and the molecule it creates is known as apolipoprotein E. What researchers have found is that there are three normal variants for the genes that code for it. In *Candle and Darkness*, Rogers compares these normal variants to the normal gene variations which produce different eye or hair color in offspring. The variations of the genes that code for this are apolipoprotein E2, E3, and E4.

The apolipoprotein E type we each have is determined by the apolipoprotein genes we inherited from each of our parents. There are actually six possible apolipoprotein E types that we can inherit including E2/E2; E2/E3; E2/E4; E3/E3; E3/E4; and E4/E4. Researchers have found that having even one E4 form of apolipoprotein E (either E2/E4 or E3/E4) increases the risk of developing Alzheimer's disease. Having a double dose of the E4 form (E4/E4) dramatically increases the risk of contracting the disease.

Geneticist Doris Zallen provides the most recent information about the risks involved in inheriting susceptibility genes in her book, *Does It Run in the Family?*. Zallen advises that the risk of developing Alzheimer's for individuals with no E4 gene by age eighty is 20 percent. Individuals with just one copy of the E4 gene have about a 45 percent chance of developing the disease. However, individuals who have inherited the two E4 genes (E4/E4) have an alarming 90 percent chance of developing the disease.[5]

To understand why the E4 form is so problematic, Rogers provides several hypotheses. One hypothesis is the relationship of apolipoprotein E to cholesterol and cardiovascular disorders. The E4 variant is associated with higher cholesterol levels, which could pose many problems, both direct and indirect, for the brain. These cholesterol problems may set the stage for Alzheimer's disease by blocking blood flow to the brain.

The other hypothesis is the one presented earlier, which describes the role of apolipoprotein E in normal cell maintenance or repair. This view holds that E4 does not fulfill what Rogers calls its "proper brain housekeeping function"[6] as well as the others, especially the most effective E2. Given the extra nerve cells we have at birth, this decreased ability to protect or repair nerve cells does not make much difference until old age. With apolipoprotein E, the loss of nerve cells occurs sooner.

Researchers are beginning to acknowledge that the genetic roots of Alzheimer's disease are present at conception. Still, according to Dr. Zallen, "this E4 variation does not deliver a knockout punch"[7] by preventing the gene or genes from functioning. Instead, the E4 variant probably brings about small changes in the way the gene carries out its function in the cell. This changed way that the gene functions may, in fact, make the victim's health more vulnerable to environmental influences. Because of the E4 influence, the altered gene may be less effective at neutralizing the toxins in the environment.

WHAT THIS MEANS TO CAREGIVERS

The complexity of susceptibility genes and "single-gene" theories with regard to Alzheimer's disease is meaningless to caregivers unless it can tell them about their risk factors. Still, for those who study Alzheimer's disease, exploring the hereditary basis of the disease not only provides hereditary information, but more importantly, genetic information can provide important clues to how the disease may be someday treated. For example, if mutations in a gene lead to Alzheimer's disease, researchers might come up with a way to dissolve the deposits. Rogers believes that further into the future, we might consider gene therapy, a scientific arena just beginning for humans, but well established for plants and animals.

With gene therapy, it has been shown that a defective gene can be replaced, or that a new gene can be added to counteract or to help. It is possible that physicians may someday be able to replace the mutated genes on chromosome 1, 14, or 21. Or, one day we may find a way to counteract the E4 variance. At present, we cannot. Still, research into the hereditary or genetic basis of the disease should eventually lead to a definitive clinical test that will diagnose Alzheimer's in living patients. By testing for genetic mutations on chromosomes, doctors can already diagnose the major forms of hereditary Alzheimer's. Doctors should also be able to test family members to determine who is likely to become a victim in the future.

Testing for a susceptibility gene such as apolipoprotein E would help in the diagnostic process. However, unlike the dominant single-gene mutation described earlier, possessing a susceptibility only confers greater risk. Researchers caution that just because you have a susceptibility gene, it does not mean that you will eventually have the disease. Fifty-five percent of those born with a single E4 gene have no signs of the disease at age eighty. Of course, 90 percent of those with a double E4 combination will indeed have the disease. Thus, a factor to consider in deciding whether to have genetic testing done is the probability of escaping the illness, even if the test results reveal the presence of E4. It is a difficult decision, and one that many families are now struggling with.

DECISIONS ABOUT GENETIC TESTING

As family caregivers to impaired parents, the day-to-day reality of the disease touches every aspect of their lives. For many, however, Alzheimer's may also touch every aspect of their future lives, well beyond the death of the impaired parent. These are the families with clear hereditary patterns of Alzheimer's. Those families with the more rare, single-gene form of it inherit the disease quite directly by inheriting a single mutant gene. There is much evidence that possessing this single-gene disorder virtually guarantees the development of early-onset Alzheimer's disease. In contrast, the more typical form of Alzheimer's disease is a late-onset disease that is primarily associated with the apolipoprotein E gene. We have already seen that the genetic predisposition associated with the possession of the E4 variation is quite substantial. Still, geneticists remind us that the predisposition associated with the E4 single gene does not represent a certainty of the disease. Most Alzheimer's disease occurs after a lifetime of exposure to all kinds of environmental influences, including stress, estrogen depletion for women, diet, and head injuries. All of these can have an influence on the risk factors. This uncertainty provides a compelling argument against testing for the susceptibility gene.

While the single-gene testing may be useful for predicting hereditary early-onset Alzheimer's, there is a strong argument to be made against testing for the presence of susceptibility genes. While useful in the diagnostic process of a person with the symptoms of Alzheimer's, the use of available testing is not encouraged for the family member without symptoms who simply wants to test for the presence of apolipoprotein E4.

There are strong arguments against testing for the gene. The first is a societal argument, the second, an even stronger individual argument. The societal argument against testing stems from concerns that Zallen presents in her book, that "genetics is not just a personal and family matter, genetic information has long been of interest to outsiders. Genetics has been used as the basis for granting insurance coverage, employment and educational opportunity to some while refusing these opportunities to others."[8] From this societal perspective, there is concern by many geneticists and ethicists that the new forms of genetic testing would be of interest to these outsiders. Geneticists question whether the genetic tests we take for personal or family reasons might be used later to discriminate against us.

Zallen reminds us that we already have examples of this societal use of genetic information from the eugenics movement of the earlier half of this century, when eugenic ideas grew into efforts to restrict immigration from southern and central Europe. These people were viewed as genetically unsound and were restricted in their entry into the United States. These restrictive quotas later had tragic consequences for people trying to escape the Nazis in the 1930s.

While it is doubtful that the United States government would ever discriminate by genetics, there remains concern that information about genes would be used by those who provide life, health, or disability insurance; or to those who provide employment or educational opportunities.

POSSIBLE DISCRIMINATION IN EMPLOYMENT

There are several opportunities for employers to use genetic testing to discriminate against workers. First, prospective job candidates may be discriminated against in hiring decisions, because the employer may be concerned that if the applicant has a gene that predisposes to Alzheimer's, he or she may be viewed as someone who will eventually have a diminished mental capacity for the position. Or employers may worry that the job applicant with the presence of a susceptibility gene for Alzheimer's would eventually become too costly for the company's health insurance plan.

These fears will most likely prove unwarranted, as there are already federal regulations against this type of discrimination in the workplace. The Americans with Disabilities Act of 1990 forbids discrimination against those with disabilities. Although possessing the susceptibility gene by itself does not render a person disabled, the law can be invoked if the individual is regarded by the employer as having an impairment. At the present time, it is a violation of the Americans with Disabilities Act to withdraw a job offer based on genetic testing. However, disabled employees may be excluded from group health insurance.

Still, there are some jobs for which strict standards demand agility, excellent judgment, and quick reaction time. For example, airplane pilots, emergency workers, police officers, and military personnel would be vulnerable. Employers in these areas may regard genetic testing as necessary to show fitness for the work, to insure the safety of others.

A second societal concern about genetic testing has to do with the availability and affordability of insurance coverage for those who have been tested.

DISCRIMINATION IN INSURANCE AVAILABILITY AND AFFORDABILITY

Insurance companies base their rates on estimates of an applicant's current and future health status. These companies already routinely do AIDS testing, EKG testing, and perform medical exams on applicants for life insurance. All of these tests are performed in an attempt to estimate the probability that the insurance companies will profit from the policy.

Current medical problems are considered "preexisting conditions," and can disqualify applicants for insurance coverage. Genetic information, if it is known, could provide insurance companies with available information about susceptibility of contracting a life-shortening disease, or one that will be costly to treat. The presence of a double E4 gene is a "preexisting condition," because it predicts a 90 percent risk of contracting Alzheimer's disease by age eighty. But for most people, age eighty is a long time in the future, and many of those who test positive for E4 will die of other causes before they even reach eighty.

Still, if insurance companies begin demanding genetic testing, they would have valuable information to enable them to discriminate against those with susceptibility genes. In anticipation of this scenario, there are now groups who are lobbying against insurance companies' ability to demand genetic testing, and to deny access to the results of tests that have already been done. Zallen points out that "if insurance companies are allowed to demand genetic testing, these companies would actually be forcing individuals to acquire information that they may had previously decided against obtaining. This would be a serious violation against the individual's right to choose against genetic testing."[9]

There are now some genetic testing insurance provisions that have been developed by some states. California and Wisconsin have broad provisions which limit insurance access to genetic test results and prohibit any use of genetic tests during the insurance application process. Other states restrict insurer access to genetic information for only a few disorders, but not Alzheimer's. At present, there are no state regulations that prevent insurers from using genetic information obtained from family history or applicant responses to questions on the medical record.

Zallen and other geneticists believe that eventually the federal government will establish a national policy for the use of genetic testing in insurance underwriting decisions. The first step toward the creation of this national policy is the 1997 Health Insurance Portability and Accountability Act. This act provides the continuance of health insurance and restricts the use of genetic information in determining eligibility for insurance.

ADDITIONAL ARGUMENTS AGAINST GENETIC TESTING

While the societal arguments against testing are strong, on a personal level they are even more compelling. The argument against genetic testing for an asymptomatic family member stems from the anxiety and possible depression that the findings might cause. Because we know that 45 percent of all who carry the single E4 gene will eventually show the symptoms of Alzheimer's disease, all who hear this diagnosis may fear that they are in fact part of the 45 percent. Even if the presence of the E4 gene may predict Alzheimer's for some, there is most likely a long time delay between when the test reveals the presence of the susceptibility gene and when the first symptoms of memory loss appear. For some, these years may become a nightmare waiting period for the earliest symptoms. Life would begin to lose meaning. Yet, we know that finding a single susceptibility gene does not mean that the corresponding illness will ever develop. By the same token, because we also know that Alzheimer's disease may occur even in the absence of the susceptibility gene, absence of E4 is no guarantee against the disease.

Still, a positive finding could lead to depression, and the patient may in fact begin to develop the memory impairment so characteristic of Alzheimer's disease. At this point, it would be unclear whether the patient is showing early-stage Alzheimer's, or whether the depression alone is causing the symptoms. We have already demonstrated that depression-related dementia arises because of the depressed person's decreased interest in life. Depressed people do not attend to conversations or events, and as a result, information is not retained. In an article for the American Psychological Association, Dr. Norman Abeles, the association's past president, believes that too often, depression combines with anxiety to become an especially potent "thought disrupter."[10] Adults with major depression can have noticeable cognitive problems. According to Abeles, these depressed people "test out" with clear memory losses, but the depression can be treated with medication or psychotherapy and the "dementia" will go away. Genetic testing could be a powerful contributor to depression and, in effect, could mimic the symptoms of Alzheimer's disease even when there is no disease present.

Still, there are others for whom the genetic testing may in fact act to relieve anxiety. Family members who are terrified of contracting the disease may look for any reassurance that they will be spared the anguish of their loved one with Alzheimer's. For them, the decision regarding testing remains complex, because a positive finding for these especially anxious family members would be traumatic.

At this time, Athena Labs, a leading Alzheimer's research company, can provide clinical tests for the presence of apolipoprotein E4, mutations in presenilin 1, or the presence or absence of neurofibrillary tangles. All of these tests can be administered using a blood sample and a cerebrospinal fluid sample. The blood test is relatively simple, but the spinal procedure to withdraw a sample of cerebrospinal fluid can be extremely painful. The test is accurate for finding signs of Alzheimer's disease about 90 percent of the time. If a presenilin mutation is found, the test will be accurate 100 percent of the time.

Still, the question remains, should concerned family members call their physicians to request a referral to Athena Labs, the testing source? Most physicians would counsel strongly against the test, unless the one requesting testing was already showing early symptoms of the disease. One of the reasons for physician reluctance is the fact that many patients without E4 or a presenilin 1 mutation still get the disease. Having these susceptibility genes only increases the risk, but cannot rule out the disease. In addition, many early-stage disease victims lack the tangle fragments in the cerebrospinal fluid. Reliability is still a problem. While a positive test for Alzheimer's can be 100 percent accurate, a negative test is only about 60 percent accurate. Physicians ordinarily do not want to recommend a test with such a high probability for the false negative finding. In these cases, the patient may believe that he or she is no longer at risk, and may not recognize what can later evolve into true symptoms of the disease.

These decisions are difficult. However, most families decide against testing since there is little that can be done, even if the susceptibility genes are present. Behavioral strategies can be helpful in managing the behaviors and improving the patient's quality of life, and some drugs have shown promise in delaying symptom onset. Still, their is nothing yet that can be done to prevent the insidious brain damage that accompanies Alzheimer's disease.

NOTES

1. Joseph Rogers, *Candle and Darkness* (Chicago, IL: Bonus Books, 1998), p. 78.

2. Rogers, *Candle and Darkness*, p. 80.

3. Rogers, *Candle and Darkness*, p. 82.

4. Rogers, *Candle and Darkness*, p. 86.

5. Doris Zallen, *Does It Run in the Family?* (New Brunswick, NJ: Rutgers University Press, 1997), p. 111.

6. Zallen, *Does It Run in the Family?*, p. 112.

7. Zallen, *Does It Run in the Family?*, p. 112.

8. Zallen, *Does It Run in the Family?*, p. 127.

9. Zallen, *Does It Run in the Family?*, p.130.

10. Marjorie Centofanti, "Fears of Alzheimer's Undermines Health of Elderly Patients," *American Psychological Association Monitor* (June 1998): p. 6.

Chapter 8

Caregiving and Quality of Life

One day at work, in what began as one of the many casual conversations with my closest colleague and friend, he surprised me with his sudden seriousness. I was describing one of the latest challenges Katharine had presented us with, and instead of one of his usual lighthearted responses, he became very serious. It was unexpected, because he has such a wonderful sense of humor. Always able to see the funny side of any situation, from the creative stories our students tell when their term papers are late yet again, to the silly stuffiness of the endless bureaucratic memos we receive, he has often helped us to see a lighter side to our heavy caregiving burden.

Because of our long history together, it was surprising to see him so serious. He knew how much our family cared about Katharine, and we had had many conversations about the ways we were responding to her, but on that Monday morning, his tone took on a quiet seriousness when he said, "If I ever get like that, I hope someone shoots me."

At first I thought he was kidding, because he often is. And his smile revealed only a halfhearted attempt at gravity. Still, his grim tone suggested that he believed it might be better to be dead than to be in what he surely thought was a miserable state like Katharine's. I began to realize that in all of my stories about Katharine, we had never talked about what the experience might be like for her. My narratives were always about our family, and our responses to her. My friend obviously had come to the conclusion that anyone who did such crazy things as Katharine must be miserable.

He was wrong about Katharine being miserable, but it was not his fault. Not once, in all of the funny "Katharine stories" did I ever tell him how much joy she still seemed to have in her life. Although we are close friends, I would not have considered bringing such serious issues to our conversations. Keeping things light provides the structure of our relationship. We often try to top each other with stories of family foibles. There is always plenty of "material" for us, as we both have teenage children and three-generation households. Plus, I had found early in our family caregiving that it is easier to smile about Katharine putting the car keys in the freezer or the soap liquid on her cereal than to constantly agonize over it. My friend had always helped me find the humor, and his daily cheerfulness has helped me on many difficult days.

On that morning, however, I realized that I never once told him that Katharine seemed happy. I never once told him that for the three years she had lived with us, she greeted me each morning with a smile and a hug. She seemed to love life as much, or maybe even more than she had loved life before her illness. She loved going for walks, petting "Charli" our fluffy Shih Tzu, and until the day she died, she loved eating chocolate ice cream. She loved looking at the flowers in the garden outside her room, and watching a bird nesting in the tree next to her window. She loved the warmth of the sun on her face, and watching the children playing at the day-care center that adjoined her own senior center. She had dozens of people at the center who loved her and constantly reminded her that she was loved. She had many pleasures in her life, and even though she could not verbally communicate much of this, I knew by the softening of her face when she saw Charli bounce into her room, that she was happy. I could sense her contentment when we would sit outside by the pool during long, sunny weekends. Katharine was happy, not in spite of the Alzheimer's disease. She was happy because after the first difficult caregiving year, her disease had progressed to the point where she no longer worried about it, or anything else.

Still, an outsider looking into Katharine's confused eyes, or trying to make sense of her garbled speech, might think that she must be miserable. It would be a mistake. But I think my friend's mistake is a common one. I am increasingly hearing his sentiments in the country's current conversations about "quality of life" concerns and "death with dignity" debates. The rhetoric which accompanied Oregon's assisted-suicide bill was filled with platitudes about "quality of life," and now these same phrases about death with dignity are creeping into California conversations surrounding a new assisted-suicide bill for the year 2000.

DEFINING QUALITY OF LIFE

Too often, people think that anyone whose cognitive ability has deteriorated must also have a deteriorating spirit. While we never can truly know what one with dementia is feeling, I can say with certainty that Katharine's dementia never prevented her from feeling love and caring. This is not to say that in the early stages of the disease, Katharine did not experience the terror of the darkness that was beginning to descend. In those early days of confusion, the horror of not knowing what was happening must have been overwhelming for her. During the early stages, Katharine did not confide her fears to anyone; her aggressiveness with strangers and would-be caretakers was certainly symptomatic of a struggling spirit.

Once the early stages had passed, however, the progressive dementia characteristic of the middle to later stages became almost a gift, because the fearfulness diminishes, and with it much of the anger. We found that these latter stages of Alzheimer's were actually the most rewarding for all of us. Katharine became progressively more confused, but the benefit was that she no longer cared that she was confused. Once again, she became happy and contented. For the caregiver, the uncertainty is over because finally, he or she truly understands the needs of the patient, the routines have developed, and the anger (for both) is gone. The mourning of the loss has most likely lessened, and the real caregiving can finally begin. During the last years of Katharine's life, a calm peacefulness finally settled over our home. Katharine was speaking very little, but she was still able to smile and respond to hugs and her favorite things.

Katharine's cognitive decline brought with it the beginnings of a physical decline. She became very unsteady on her feet, and progressed from a cane to a walker to help her ambulate. Eventually, she no longer was able to figure out how to use her walker without help. We added wheels to the walker, and when Katharine was standing up and steady, we would position her hands on the bars and pull the center bar to kind of pull her along. Certainly, there were new challenges, but these were minor compared with the early stages of confusion when she was a whirlwind of crazy activity. The dozens of door and closet locks were no longer necessary because Katharine had neither the ability nor the motivation to try and "go home."

Katharine was now incontinent and had difficulty feeding herself. Finger foods became her meals; we simply would cut up bite-sized pieces of sandwiches or soft meats and place them on a TV tray. She was no longer eating with us at the dining room table, but she always had company. Whenever he was home, Dana began sitting with her while she ate, and mealtime became her favorite part of the day. At that point, she was still able to smile, and her face beamed when Dana was with her for her meals.

In fact, one of the greatest gifts of this late stage in our caregiving was the opportunity for Dana to once again take a more active role in caregiving. No longer afraid of Dana as a stranger, and no longer making demands to go home, Katharine was again a joy for him. He was finally able to enjoy spending time with her. She was still able to attend day care—the wonderful staff at Glenner had assured us that they were happy to tend to the growing number of physical and emotional needs of their loving charges. On Saturday mornings, Dana began driving Katharine to day care, and picking her up each Saturday afternoon. It gave me a welcome one-day break from my daily day-care chauffeuring routine.

Looking back now, we are all grateful the we had this opportunity to care for Katharine in these final stages, because we were truly caregiving at that point, not simply providing a locked facility in our home. We would not have wanted to miss this time. For us, it became a reminder of who Katharine truly was. We talked about it often, realizing that the later-stage caring created an opportunity for us once again to appreciate her. We had almost forgotten the Katharine we used to know, and these late stages helped us remember. In some ways, the essence of Katharine was again visible to us once the anxiety and restlessness of the early stages had passed. A theologian might say that this time of caregiving became for us, an affirmation of Katharine's soul. The struggle was over, and the caregiving was truly caring.

CAREGIVING AS AFFIRMATION OF THE SOUL

When my friend told me of his end-of-life worries, I would have liked to talk about Katharine's soul. But he, with his Ivy League Ph.D., and I, with my quiet Catholicism, tend to remain silent on these issues. Soul-talk is not something we do, even with close friends, especially funny close friends. Still, I might have liked to talk with him of what Christians believe from faith—that it is the notion of the soul that is fundamental to personal identity. I would have liked to tell him that Katharine was still Katharine because her soul remained throughout life, even after the disappearance of her conscious, knowing self.

A recent book on mortality by M. Scott Peck, entitled *Denial of the Soul*, reminds us that for those with faith, there is the knowledge that the soul of the individual remains, even in dementia.[1] Because the essence or soul of Katharine remained, she was beloved still as a mother, a mother-in-law, a grandmother, and most importantly, as a child of God. She was still Katharine, even when she remembered nothing of herself. She no longer even recognized her own reflection in the mirror, but we remembered, and we tried to remind her often of how much she was loved. Although Katharine did not know who she was, we certainly did. We began to realize that we were caring for the soul of Katharine, even though at the very end of her life, we seemed only to be meeting her needs for warmth, food, rest, and loving touch. On the surface, she no longer seemed to be Katharine, because her behaviors, her speech, and even her mannerisms were so different from the woman we had always known. Yet, we certainly knew that her soul was most definitely Katharine. And there were glimmers of Katharine throughout the entire time she lived with us.

In his book, *Forgetting Whose We Are*, David Keck calls Alzheimer's the "theological disease" because although the disease may ravage the body, he maintains that it does nothing to affect the soul.[2] We, too, are fortunate to have had so many friends who reminded us of the grace that comes from caregiving. Our priest, who had become acquainted with Katharine during our early caregiving days when we were still bringing her to mass each week, reminded us often of the grace that God gives to caregivers.

For those without faith, however, when Alzheimer's disease peels away the identity of the person, there is little left but despair. In the case described below, the husband of an Alzheimer's-impaired woman said that his wife wanted to end her life before "it became peeled away, layer by layer, until there was nothing." His words deny the existence of her soul.[3]

EUTHANASIA AS DENIAL OF THE SOUL

For those who work with Alzheimer's disease patients, it was especially saddening that the premiere performance of Dr. Jack Kevorkian's suicide machine (which he invented for the assisted suicide of the terminally ill) would be used by someone like Janet Adkins, an early-stage Alzheimer's sufferer. News stories reported that on a hot summer day in 1990, in a Detroit campground, Janet Adkins was the first to find herself reclining on a metal cot in the back of that now-famous rusted old Volkswagen van. We learned that she was attended by a doctor who hooked her up to a heart monitor, slid an intravenous needle into a vein in her arm, and began a saline solution flowing through the tube. Within moments, the news reports claimed, the doctor instructed Mrs. Adkins to push a big red button at the base of the machine.[4] A compliant, early-stage Alzheimer's victim, Mrs. Adkins was quite willing to do what she was told to do, even if she had little idea of the full and final consequences of her actions. Immediately, the saline was replaced by a pain killer; one minute later, the poisonous potassium chloride began to flow; and within the next few minutes, Janet Adkins became the first and most famous recipient of the services of Dr. Jack Kevorkian. It was now official—Dr. Kevorkian's first assisted suicide was an Alzheimer's patient.

Many in the Alzheimer's caregiving community asked, how could this act be termed a suicide? Anyone who truly understands Alzheimer's disease knows that its very diagnosis posits a severely impaired judgment and an inability to make rational decisions. Even in the early stages, there is a profound lack of awareness of the consequences of one's behavior. And, in these early days of the disease, because of the growing confusion and loss of ability, there is often severe depression. Still, Kevorkian spent the next few months on a media tour, with appearances on *Geraldo, Nightline, Oprah,* and the usual television news programs, proudly proclaiming that Adkins made her decision competently. Adkins's diagnosis belies this assertion. Caregivers know that the diagnosis of Alzheimer's is completely incompatible with Kevorkian's claims of competence in decision making. The major symptom of Alzheimer's disease is sufficient mental deterioration to impair the ability to make decisions. Therefore, Mrs. Adkins would not have been diagnosed with Alzheimer's disease if her judgment and decision-making ability had not been impaired.

Yet, some euthanasia advocates continue to call Dr. Kevorkian "a brave pioneer." He describes his device as "humane, dignified, and painless,"[5] and he insists that his critics are "brainwashed ethicists and religious nuts." On his many television appearances, Kevorkian portrays himself as a modern prophet confronting doctors' hypocrisy and society's misunderstanding of death. He was quoted as saying that "the law and ethics flatly don't mean a thing to me when a patient is in front of me and needs help." Kevorkian claims never to have had a doubt about helping Adkins die before Alzheimer's made her life unbearable.

He believes that he was the ultimate humanitarian. Mrs. Adkins's husband said that he, too, was convinced that his wife was determined to die. The Adkins family had heard about the suicide machine after Kevorkian received national notoriety and demonstrated his invention for the media. Once Janet Adkins had been diagnosed with Alzheimer's, she contacted Kevorkian, sent him her clinical records, and was chosen to be the first to use the new machine.

At the time of the assisted suicide, there was little societal criticism about the fact that Kevorkian's first victim was an Alzheimer's patient. The fact that Adkins had Alzheimer's disease probably made her especially attractive to Kevorkian, because he knew of the terror that a diagnosis of Alzheimer's can inspire in others. He must have known that many would agree that Alzheimer's is indeed a disease that calls for a consideration of euthanasia. And, as expected, few of the news reports even remarked on the choice of an early-stage Alzheimer's patient as being appropriate for the machine. The fact that Adkins had played tennis the day before she was put to death was incidental. Her tennis playing was used as "evidence" that she was competent in her decision making. Anyone who has worked with Alzheimer's patients knows, however, that there are many behaviors that the Alzheimer's patient can continue and enjoy, including golf, tennis, and even swimming—without possessing the higher functioning skills to actually know exactly what he or she is doing.

For Adkins, the criticism focused instead upon the use of the rusty van for the deadly work. Kevorkian's response was revealing, as he angrily stated in an interview: "Where was Christ born? The world's worst conditions, in a haystack with manure and animals all around."[6] This is a revealing analogy from a man who seems to have taken on the role of God.

Still, there are many who agree with his mission and seek him out for his services. The Klooster family introduced in chapter 2 is a good example. In the bitter family custody trial, testimony showed Mrs. Klooster, the wife of the Alzheimer's patient, as having written several letters to Kevorkian. She signed one letter requesting assisted suicide, that was supposedly narrated by her severely demented husband, with an "X" because he was too impaired to even sign his own name. The suicide was prevented only because Mr. Klooster's son rescued his father from Dr. Kevorkian. The 911 call made by Mrs. Klooster demanding that something be done about her son's kidnapping of his father revealed an irate woman, saying: "My son kidnapped my husband. He can't have him, he belongs to me." In fact, this has been Mrs. Klooster's strongest argument throughout the sad case—that her husband "belongs" to her, and she knows that death is what would have been best for him.

For Mrs. Klooster, Mr. Adkins, and others, there is the belief that Alzheimer's is nothing more than a "slow death" in which the person disappears and there is nothing left. When Mr. Adkins says that his wife wanted to end her life before "it became peeled away, layer by layer, until there was nothing," his words reveal his belief that when the conscious self is gone, there is nothing at the core. With this belief, options of ending a dimming life become possible. And, increasingly, Alzheimer's patients' families are looking at these options.

Their search for a release from the caregiving is understandable. There were many times in the early days of our caregiving that I was certainly ready to abandon the work. Our lives seemed out of control, and we had no idea when we would ever get back to normal. Worse, I knew that Katharine felt out of control in those early days, when her confusion worsened and her family began making decisions for her. I am grateful, though, that we never allowed our need for control over the course of her disease to guide our decisions; for some, this need leads to unspeakable acts.

MERCY KILLING BY THE CAREGIVER

Perhaps what is most dangerous about a culture that seems to support euthanasia, is the encouragement that it appears to give to those desperate few caregivers who choose to end the lives of their loved ones by themselves. In 1995, Jean Brush, an obviously overwhelmed caregiver to her eighty-one-year-old Alzheimer's-impaired husband, murdered him by stabbing. Exhausted by the caregiving demands, Mrs. Brush's defense maintained that she killed her husband to end his suffering. She described his life as "tortured and filled with hallucinations."[7] Outside, he saw threatening armies marching down the street. To him, neighbors' cars violently shook back and forth; electrical wires lay strewn around the house; and water gushed from holes in the bedroom ceiling, drenching his bed. When his wife tried to reassure him that he was only seeing things, Mr. Brush accused her of being part of a conspiracy. He thought she had a contract with someone to torture him.

Mrs. Brush says she "helped" her husband end his life, and, it would appear that the Canadian judge agreed with her. She narrated to the judge that she was unable to find a placement in a nursing home for him. He was on a waiting list for a placement when she led him into the dining room of their home, laid him on some blankets she had draped across the floor, and proceeded to stab him to death with a five-inch hunting knife. Judge Bernd Zabel called her actions "a desperate attempt to end her husband's life with some dignity."[8]

Most readers might question whether being stabbed to death on the dining room floor by one's wife qualifies as a death with dignity. Yet, despite the violence of the crime, Zabel gave her a suspended sentence with eighteen months probation. This meant that Mrs. Brush would not serve any time in prison. Zabel stated that, "She has already suffered a harsher sentence than could ever be imposed on her life, the loss of her loving husband."[9]

This is not the only case in which caregivers to Alzheimer's disease have murdered their loved ones and received no punishment. This is a problem because by failing to punish perpetrators of these crimes, society is actually sanctioning euthanasia in cases of Alzheimer's disease. This case, like the Klooster and Adkins cases, are all examples of families "knowing" what their loved one would want, and attempting to control the course of the disease. It is a worrisome trend, and one that is related to a growing need for autonomy in our lives.

ALZHEIMER'S AND AUTONOMY

Many who write about Alzheimer's disease believe that what seems so frightening about the disease is the realization of the loss of control over our lives. This fear is what my friend was referring to when he said he would want someone to end his life before he became like Katharine. This fear about a loss of autonomy is what seems to drive the discussions on quality of life, death with dignity, and the growing euthanasia movement. We fear the loss of control, and increasingly, we are trying to find a way to control these losses, or at least cut the losses. Those with concerns about control seem to have plenty of help from a growing assisted-suicide movement that holds out the promise of not only the ability to control the end of our lives, but also the right to do so.

In a disturbingly persuasive book entitled *Life's Dominion*, philosopher Ronald Dworkin presents a strong argument for what he calls "an integrity view of autonomy"[10] in making end-of-life decisions for terminally ill patients. For Dworkin, integrity in autonomy holds that we all have a sense of the style of life we think is appropriate, and that we made choices during our lives to support this style of life. Dworkin writes that choosing death is a way to express and, "vividly confirm the values" that we believe have been most important to our lives. He believes that the integrity view of autonomy will grant freedom for people to act in ways that are keeping with their values. Those who have valued autonomy throughout their lives, should be allowed autonomy in choices surrounding death.

While some may find in Dworkin's work a compelling argument in favor of euthanasia for the patient who is rationally exercising his or her autonomy in choosing death, the argument fails when it is applied to a patient with dementia. Dworkin acknowledges the difficulty of choosing death for a demented person. His chapter entitled "Life Past Reason" focuses upon the question of what moral rights people in the late stages of dementia retain, and, what is best for them. He asks whether mentally incapacitated people have the same rights as normally competent people, or whether demented people's rights are altered or diminished in some way because of their disease. He asks, "do they, for example, have the same rights to autonomy, to the care of their custodians, to dignity, and to a minimum level of resources as sick people of normal mental competence?" Dworkin believes that they do, and most would agree, but he extends these rights to the right to end their lives, if they do so with integrity, or in keeping with the way they would have chosen death during their rational lives.

To illustrate his point, Dworkin provides the reader with a case study of an Alzheimer's patient named Margo, which was first published by Andrew Firlik in 1991, in the *Journal of the American Medical Association*. Firlik was a medical student when he met fifty-five-year old Margo, and began visiting her daily in her apartment, where she was cared for by an attendant. Like our Alzheimer's-proofed home, Margo's apartment had many locks to keep her from slipping out at night and wandering, as she had done in the past. Each time Firlik would visit, Margo said she knew who he was, but she never used his name. He suspected that this was just politeness. She told him she was reading mysteries, but Firlik noted that her place in the book jumped randomly from day to day. He thought that maybe she felt good just sitting and humming to herself, rocking back and forth, slowly nodding off, and occasionally turning to a fresh page. Firlik states that he was confused by the fact that "despite her illness, or maybe somehow because of it, Margo is undeniably one of the happiest people I have ever known." [11] He reports particularly, her pleasure at eating peanut butter and jelly sandwiches. Like the other Alzheimer's patients in her art therapy class, Firlik writes that Margo painted the same image day after day: a drawing of four circles, in soft rosy colors, one inside the other. Firlik found something graceful about the degeneration of her mind, leaving her carefree, always cheerful. He asks: "Do her problems, whatever she may perceive them to be, simply fail to make it to the worry centers of her brain?" He then asks: "When a person can no longer accumulate new memories as the old rapidly fade, what remains? Who is Margo?" Firlik suggests that her drawing of circles represented Margo's expression of her mind, her identity, and that by repeating the drawing, she was reminding herself and others of that identity. For him, the painting was Margo, "plain and contained, smiling in her peaceful demented state."[12]

In *Life's Dominion*, however, Dworkin asks the reader to look at Margo's rights and interests in two different ways: as a demented person, emphasizing her present situation and capacities; or as a person who has become demented, having an eye to the course of her whole life. If we look, as he believes we should, at the latter, Dworkin asks whether a competent person's right to autonomy includes the power to dictate that life-prolonging treatment be denied him later, or that funds not be spent on maintaining him in great comfort, even if he, when demented, demands it. For Dworkin this is especially important if these current desires are not in keeping with the demented person's previous wishes.

To illustrate, Dworkin asks the reader to imagine that the now cheerful and contented Margo may have (years ago, when fully competent) executed a formal document directing that if she should develop dementia, she should not receive treatment for any other serious, life-threatening disease she might contract; or, that when she developed dementia, she should be killed as soon and as painlessly as possible.

Under these circumstances, Dworkin provides a philosophical argument for giving support to Margo's prior wishes to end her life, despite the happiness and value she seems to now be experiencing in her dementia. Like my colleague, who half-jokingly says that he would want someone to shoot him if he became demented, Dworkin argues that Margo should be killed, even though she is content and happy in her demented state. His argument in favor of killing Margo is based on her rational wish prior to her dementia. Dworkin arrives at this position of choosing death for a demented individual by drawing upon the values of autonomy, beneficence, and dignity. He argues that a person who has become demented retains his critical interests, because what happens to him then affects the value or success of his life as a whole. He says that this decision to end his life would be in keeping with choices made when rational: "That he remains a person and that the overall value of his life continues to be intrinsically important, are decisive truths in favor of his right to dignity."[13]

Dworkin affirms that by meeting the demented person's wishes to end his life, "we mark his continued moral standing and affirm the importance of the life he has lived, by insisting that nothing be done to, or for him that denies him dignity." For Dworkin, "this is proof of the dominating grip of the idea that human life has intrinsic as well as personal importance for human beings, the complex but inescapable idea that it is sacred."

Dworkin's argument may be compelling for some, but his assertion that killing someone who is obviously happy and content is proof of the sacredness of life does not make sense to most who care for those with Alzheimer's disease. The argument fails because it is inherently a contradiction—taking life can never affirm its sacredness.

A SOCIOLOGICAL ARGUMENT AGAINST EUTHANASIA

Director of the Hastings Center, Daniel Callahan asserts that euthanasia can never be classified as a private matter of self-determination, or as an autonomous act of managing one's private affairs. Callahan posits that "euthanasia is a social decision."[14] It involves the one to be killed, the one doing the killing, and it requires a compliant society to make it acceptable. For these reasons, Callahan believes that euthanasia must be assessed in its social dimensions.

For Callahan, and an increasing number of ethicists, Dworkin's appeal to autonomy to justify euthanasia for one individual does not adequately account for the social dimensions of that individual act, nor the impact that sanctioning euthanasia as a practice will have on the common good.

The common good argument reminds us that the way we die is important not only to us, but to society at large. A society that would encourage families to kill their demented loved ones will have an enormous impact on our beliefs about our health care delivery system. Euthanasia may be viewed by patients, families, and physicians as a possible solution to our growing concerns about diminishing Medicare dollars, as a way to save scarce health care monies for more worthy cases. The elderly are already less likely to have access to lifesaving procedures than the nonelderly, and a recent study has documented that the elderly receive far fewer diagnostic procedures and emergency treatments.

In his book on moral theology and euthanasia, Richard Gula creates a powerful argument against euthanasia from the perspective of the common good. Like Callahan, his sociologically and theologically grounded argument is based on the conviction that there is a good for society as a whole beyond a good for each person. He states that: "The common good respects and serves the interests of individuals, the common good ultimately upholds the collective good as more important than the good of any one individual."[15] Respect for the common good posits that the individual will flourish only as far as society as a whole flourishes. To seek the common good is to seek those actions and policies that would contribute to the total well-being of persons and the community.

While a strong argument, the common good debate has not met with success. Gula suggests that one of the reasons for the lack of success in the euthanasia controversy is that the diversity of society makes it difficult for all to appreciate that there can indeed be some good that is of value to us as a whole, irrespective of our differences. He writes that, "As long as we continue to envision society as a loose association of diverse individuals bound together by self-interest, then we will continue to miss the value of the common good."[16]

It is also possible that the reason the common good argument has not been embraced is the continuing value we place on our independence. When President Reagan was diagnosed with Alzheimer's disease, it must have been difficult for such a strong individual, such a seemingly independent man, to cope with the loss of autonomy. The image of the healthy Reagan, in part created by his early films and by the media in his campaign ads, was that of a rugged outdoor cowboy. We often saw him pictured on his horse, or mending fences and clearing brush around his California retreat in the hills. The image was certainly one of an individualist.

Beyond the image, though, the reality of many of his decisions throughout his presidency reflected his independence. Often taking unpopular stands and battling the opposition, he showed remarkable courage. This courage was again evident in his good-bye letter to the nation, when he spoke of his sadness over his inability to protect his loving wife from having to take care of him now. Still, in his letter, he also said that he would continue to fight. While it was clear that he mourned the loss of autonomy, he also was able to surrender it when needed. It was also evident that he would continue to fight the battle with Alzheimer's with integrity. His respect for life was demonstrated in the policies he supported throughout his tenure. A life of integrity for Reagan has meant to continue to provide an example of a life with dignity, despite the disease.

President Reagan and his family's dignified response to Alzheimer's is a reminder of something I have learned in our caregiving experiences, and in my work with caregivers and dementia patients. The way we respond to the diagnosis of Alzheimer's disease simply reflects the person we have become up to that point. How we will cope is a matter of what we have come to believe about life, the values we hold, and the attitudes we take. If we have lived a life of love and dignity, we will accept the diagnosis similarly. If we have not already developed the "habits of the heart" to enable us to live this life, we will not have the dignity to help us in death. Callahan reminds us that "How we die will be an expression of how we have wanted to live, and the meaning we have found in our dying will be at one with the meaning we have found in our living."[17]

From this perspective, the euthanasia and assisted suicide movement is as much a challenge to our depth of moral character as it is a challenge to the meaning of our moral principles. Gula asserts that,

As mortal persons, we must face the fact that life is inevitably marked by illness, aging, decline and death. The humble person knows that reality will ultimately go its own way and follow its own internal dynamism. To die with dignity, the humble do not have to be in charge of the interior self so as to integrate into life, the unexpected as well as the unwanted circumstances of life. Acquiring the virtue of humility as a desirable goal is one step towards making euthanasia something we could not even imagine.[18]

Gula's sociological perspective is strengthened by his spiritual perspective, which appeals to a combination of the principles of divine sovereignty and human stewardship. From a spiritual perspective, he argues that human life is God's gift to us for which we are responsible. This attitude of reverence is enshrined in the principle of sanctity of life. From this perspective, human life is not properly reverenced by putting others at the disposal of whims, ambitions, or desires to serve some utilitarian end.

Still, as the following will show, there is increasing evidence that we seem to be moving far from humility and reverence for life—in Oregon, in the Netherlands, and California is also again moving in this direction.

GROWING SUPPORT FOR ASSISTED SUICIDE

In 1994, Oregon voters passed Ballot Measure 16, a measure to allow Oregon citizens access to physician-assisted suicide. Exit polls revealed that voters clearly believed that those in horrible pain should be allowed to end their suffering. Likewise, a challenge to Measure 16 in 1997 failed to repeal the bill. We are now beginning to learn about the outcomes of this legislation.

A recent study published in the *New England Journal of Medicine* reveals that the outcome of assisted suicide in Oregon is not at all close to what most voters believed would happen regarding the purpose of alleviating pain and suffering of the terminally ill. The article reported that of the fifteen individuals who legally committed suicide with the assistance of their doctors in 1998, not one of them was forced into the assisted suicide because of their intractable pain or suffering. Instead, each person had strong personal beliefs in individual autonomy, and chose suicide based primarily on fears of future dependence. These individuals did not want to lose their ability to control their lives. The article also reported that the people who received assisted suicide had comparatively shorter relationships with their doctors than those who died naturally. The first woman to commit assisted suicide in Oregon had a two-week relationship with the doctor who assisted her. Her personal physician refused to help her, as did a second doctor who diagnosed her with depression. The woman went to an assisted-suicide advocacy group, which referred her to a physician willing to provide the lethal dosage. This woman was not atypical, as the study demonstrates that six of the fifteen people sought assistance from two or more doctors.[19]

Oregon's frightening findings are given more meaning when coupled with results from a study of euthanasia in the Netherlands. While there are two Dutch penal codes which make both assisted suicide and euthanasia illegal, the reality is that doctors who directly euthanize patients or help patients kill themselves will not be prosecuted as long as they follow certain guidelines, including reporting every euthanasia/assisted suicide to the local prosecutors. In 1991, the results of the first official government study of the practice of Dutch euthanasia was released. The data demonstrate that despite long-standing, court-approved euthanasia guidelines developed to protect patients, abuse has become the norm. According to the government-sponsored Remmelink Report, in one year (1990): 2,300 people died as the result of doctor-initiated euthanasia; 400 people died as a result of doctors providing them with the means to kill themselves through assisted suicide; and an alarming 1,040 (an average three patients per day during all of 1990) died from involuntary euthanasia. Follow-up studies indicated that in one out of five euthanasia cases (nearly 1,000 euthanasia cases per year), the patient had not asked to be euthanized. This means that doctors actively performed euthanasia on these patients without their knowledge or consent. Of this latter group, 14 percent of those involuntarily killed were fully competent, and 72 percent had never given any indication that they would want to end their lives. Most chilling, in 45 percent of the cases involving hospitalized patients who were involuntarily euthanized, the patients' families had no knowledge that their loved ones' lives were deliberately terminated by doctors.[20]

The Dutch findings are contrary to the right-to-die rhetoric, which holds that euthanasia and assisted suicide are "choice issues." The data clearly demonstrate that where euthanasia and assisted suicide are accepted practice, patients have little choice at all. Alzheimer's victims and their families have serious concerns in the Netherlands, and they should have serious concerns here, also.

When trying to understand why Oregon is at the frontier of the assisted-suicide movement, it is important to note that the states's rates of church attendance and membership are among the lowest in the nation. Actually, Oregon's rates are second only to Alaska. Fewer than 10 percent of all Oregon residents are members of the Catholic Church, the leading opponent of the 1994 initiative, and Oregon residents are among the least likely people in the country to view issues through the filter of religious guidance. This lack of regard for religious teachings, coupled with the rugged individualistic philosophy still strong in the West, prevents them from appreciating even the sociological argument for the common good.

Concerns are growing in California, as caregivers are becoming alarmed that the pro-choice rhetoric of Oregon is once again reaching voters in their state. California, an even larger western state, may come closer to passing the assisted suicide bill this time. The success of this initiative is given even more support when the individualist arguments are coupled with economic arguments. In a state like California, the economic argument may be persuasive to some because of ever-dwindling health care resources for an ever-expanding population of uninsured citizens. If assisted suicide became legally sanctioned in California, some might be encouraged to choose to end their lives rather than take the chance of being an expensive burden to their families. Alzheimer's victims may have the decision made for them.

NOTES

1. M. Scott Peck, *Denial of the Soul* (New York: Harmony Books, 1997).

2. David Keck, *Forgetting Whose We Are* (Nashville, TN: Abingdon Press, 1996), p. 15.

3. G. Borger, "The Odd Odyssey of Dr. Death," *U.S. News and World Report* (August 27, 1990): p. 27.

4. N. Gibbs and M. McBride, "Dr. Death's Suicide Machine," *Time* (June 18, 1990): p. 69.

5. "Equals Murder?" *The Economist* (December 15, 1990): p. 28.

6. Borger, "The Odd Odyssey of Dr. Death," p. 28.

7. Scott Steele, "Mercy Killing," *Macleans* (March 13, 1995): p. 32.

8. Steele, "Mercy Killing," p. 34.

9. Steele, "Mercy Killing," p. 35.

10. Ronald Dworkin, *Life's Dominion: An Argument about Abortion, Euthanasia and Individual Freedom* (New York: Alfred A. Knopf, 1993).

11. Andrew Firlik, "Margo's Logo," *Journal of the American Medical Association* (1991): p. 201.

12. Firlik, "Margo's Logo," p. 202.

13. Cited in Rebecca Dresser, "Dworkin on Dementia" *Hastings Center Report* (November/December 1995): p. 32.

14. Daniel Callahan, "When Self-Determination Runs Amok," *Hastings Center Report* 22 (March/April 1992): pp. 52–55.

15. Richard Gula, *Euthanasia: Moral and Pastoral Perspectives* (Mahweh, NJ: Paulist Press, 1994), p. 14.

16. Gula, *Euthanasia*, p. 18.

17. Daniel Callahan, *The Troubled Dream of Life* (New York: Touchstone Books, 1993), p. 149.

18. Gula, *Euthanasia*, p. 52.

19. Arthur Chin, Katrina Hedberg, Grant Higginson, and David Fleming, "Legalized Assisted Suicide in Oregon, The First Year's Experience," *The New England Journal of Medicine* 340 (February 18, 1999).

20. Remmelink Report (The Hague: Edo Uitgeverij, 1991). Translated later by the Hemlock Society, "Euthanasia and Assisted Suicide by General Practitioners in the Netherlands" (undated publication). The Hastings Center has released several publications describing Dutch practices of euthanasia and assisted suicide, including Maurice A. M. de Wachter, "Euthanasia in the Netherlands," *Hastings Center Report* 22 (March/April 1992): pp. 23–30. Also, Daniel Callahan's *Troubled Dream of Life* presents an overview of the Remmelink Report, pp. 112–116.

Chapter 9

✳

The Caregiving Journey Ends

Many Alzheimer's caregivers' lives become sidetracked—friendships, activities, club memberships, and sometimes, even careers are suspended. Family vacations are postponed, family weddings and anniversary celebrations are missed, birthday parties are cancelled, and children's and grandchildren's graduations often go unattended.

For us, the greatest loss occurred during that difficult first caregiving year. My own mother was diagnosed with cancer, and died within the year. I wasn't there to help; my sisters and father graciously assumed all of the caregiving. They never complained that I was not there to help during the final painful days. Their loving caregiving, coupled with Hospice support, allowed my mother to stay in her Connecticut home until she died. They always reassured me that they understood I had to stay in San Diego with Katharine, but I know it was difficult for them. Both of my sisters work full-time and have families of their own. Hospice workers greatly eased the burden for them, but I know that they would have appreciated my help. I was unhappy to have missed being there.

There is always sadness and loss that accompanies caregivers' lives. The costs of protracted caregiving are high for everyone in the family in terms of the emotional toll extracted from disturbed family relationships, absentee parenting, or work-family conflicts. In addition to these emotional costs, financial costs can quickly deplete a family's resources.

Homes are often remortgaged, life insurance policies liquidated, and even college tuition funds for children or grandchildren may be spent on caregiving expenses.

Because of the overwhelming toll on the caregiving family, it is understandable that many might welcome any relief from the burden of the caregiving. Nursing home placements hold out the promise of relief, yet the reality remains that while these facilities can transfer the burden from the home, they can never transfer the burden from the heart of the caregiver. For these caregivers, the heart continues to ache each day, as they watch a loved one fade away. Day after day, in nursing homes throughout the country, the nobility and loyalty of a beloved spouse, or a devoted child is witnessed at countless Alzheimer's sufferers' bedsides.

There is a weariness in many of the caregiver's faces I have seen during the past three years. The weariness is there in the faces of the support group participants. It is also there in the faces at the bedsides, revealing a tired spirit as well as a tired body. But for these caregivers, there is the pain of not really knowing what the loved one is feeling or thinking. I remember wondering what Katharine's dreams were like. I worried that as she slept she might be frightened by the images she saw in her dreams. There is always the belief that life cannot truly resume until the death of their beloved Alzheimer's-inflicted spouse or parent. It is a painful realization, because it brings with it great ambivalence, as they know that wishing for the death of a loved one is never acceptable. Yet, the caregiver's own dreams, like mine, are often filled with thoughts of escape.

During our own early caregiving days, I remember spending time trying to identify exactly when Katharine developed Alzheimer's disease. When I wrote that my husband and I used to spend hours looking through family photo albums trying to determine when Katharine began to show the symptoms, I declined to mention that the real reason for my attempt at dating the onset of the illness was to try to determine the length of it. In those early days, I was silently computing how much longer she might live, and guiltily longing for the days when our lives might begin again. I was a frequent visitor to confession in those early days.

Conflicted wishes for a release from the caregiving were an everyday occurrence for all of us during that first year. I know that we were not alone in these wishes; support group participants often speak of their guilt when they realize that they too are hoping for death to put an end to the unending caregiving. As we have seen throughout this book, there are cases when loved ones feel so desperate that they actually kill their Alzheimer's-afflicted spouse or parent.

This would not happen if they might have been able to find help during the difficult days. For some families, Hospice can be a valued resource. However, we were told by Katharine's physicians that although the disease was indeed terminal, her death was not imminent, and she would not qualify for Hospice. Hospice care is designed to assist families in the final six months of life, and for an Alzheimer's patient, the final days are often years away.

Still, there are some fortunate Alzheimer's families who have benefited greatly from the extraordinary support that Hospice can provide. In some parts of the country, and for some Hospice providers, the six-month rule appears to be more flexible. In many ways, Hospice helps the families of the Alzheimer's patients even more than the patients themselves. While the goal of Hospice is comfort care for the patient, their services to families are invaluable. My father and sisters continue to be grateful for the loving care they all received from the Hospice nurses assigned to assist my mother. Late-stage Alzheimer's patients' families have had similar experiences.

We never felt the need for Hospice care because Katharine was so healthy and once the first difficult caregiving year had passed, the days in our household became almost easy. We began to actually see some of the benefits and joys of the caregiving. It became difficult to even remember the harried early caregiving days as the security of routines had developed, peace was restored, and our lives once again took on many of the predictable routines we had enjoyed before Katharine moved in with us.

Day care had created for all of us, a peaceful respite from the disease. Katharine's days were filled with friends at the Alzheimer's center, pets, gardens, safe outdoor walks, and a loving and affectionate day-care staff who provided her with activities to keep her challenged and entertained all day. Medication had not been needed in nearly two years. She was once again engaged in life and was adding meaning to ours.

Certainly, this is not to say that caregiving became easy. As the disease progressed, there were new tasks to be added every few weeks, but eventually even the new tasks became routine, as they too became integrated into the rhythm of the day. Our days were always full, sometimes exhausting, but never stressful, because we had finally learned to manage what needed to be done.

Once we had developed our routine of home caregiving and day care, with the invaluable day-care support network we had been fortunate to be able to build, there was never a day when we would have even considered sending Katharine to live elsewhere. Life was finally manageable, and we all were back in control of our lives. Katharine was happy, and Jonathan was enjoying seventh grade without the stresses at home that he had endured the first year.

Christmas was especially joyous during that third year. Because Katharine was again enjoying being a part of our activities, we were finally confident in inviting friends to our home. For the first time in three Christmas seasons, we had a Christmas party. Our Christmas card to relatives and closest family friends showed a family picture with Katharine sitting by our Christmas tree with Charli, her favorite pet, perched contentedly on her lap. We began to think that we could continue the caregiving forever.

Of course, as all caregivers to those with Alzheimer's know, there is nothing predictable about the disease. Just when we thought we were prepared for everything, Katharine began to slip. At first, we were sure she had a cold. She was pale and her energy was waning. As she walked from her first-floor bedroom to our car each morning on our way to day care, I noticed that her breathing had become slightly labored, and that she was becoming more unsteady than usual. The ever-vigilant day-care staff had also noticed that Katharine was tiring more easily. While her appetite was still excellent, she no longer seemed able to go on the neighborhood walks with the day-care friends and staff. A few days later, she was unable to even participate in the sing-alongs and the crafts that she had grown to love.

Katharine clearly was failing, but neither the day-care workers nor I worried, because we assumed that it was most likely the natural progression of the disease. I was sure that she was experiencing a common component of the late-stage muscle weaknesses associated with Alzheimer's. I had always known that the disease would progress to the point where eventually she would be unable to walk. I began to dread that we were beginning to approach that point.

Unfortunately, the weakness became dramatically worse. An alarmed day-care staff advised us that this was no longer a natural progression of the disease; they knew that a drastic change in condition is not often associated with Alzheimer's. This disease causes a gradual, almost imperceptible decline, unlike the dramatic weakening we were witnessing. We began to realize that Katharine was seriously ill. I made an appointment with her doctor for the following morning.

By the next day, Katharine was unable to even get out of bed without help. Unable to walk, she would not be able to get to the car to keep the doctor's appointment. I considered calling for an ambulance, but recalled that Katharine's previous two visits to the emergency room had been traumatic. While well-intentioned and respectful, on both occasions, the emergency personnel tried to deal with her in a rational and perfunctory way. Even though I told them that Katharine had Alzheimer's disease, the emergency room staff persistently tried to explain complex procedures and directions to her. They tried rushing her, and expected her to understand and obey their instructions. On both previous emergency room visits, Katharine had become combative. On our final visit, when Katharine had seizures, they placed her in restraints.

The two hospital visits taught us that an emergency room was not a safe place for a severely demented Alzheimer's patient. It was unfair to the already overburdened emergency room personnel, who need to tend to acutely ill people, and most importantly, it was unfair to put Katharine through that confusion. Still, the fact remained that Katharine needed immediate medical attention.

When I called her physician's office to explain my transportation dilemma, the sympathetic office manager told me about a new service to the elderly that a physician group in neighboring Point Loma had begun to offer. The young office manager said, without a trace of irony, that the new service was called "house calls." While I was certainly old enough to recall that doctors had made house calls in the past, this young woman had never even heard of them before the creation of the "new service." She had no idea that just a few decades ago, doctors had routinely visited patients in their homes. House calls were ended when doctors convinced us that visiting the office was necessary to enable us to benefit from the advanced technology that awaited us there.

Ironically, it is the advances in technology that are once again allowing doctors, who are so inclined, to make house calls. The competent and caring doctor who visited Katharine on that rainy February Friday afternoon brought an arsenal of technology, in miniature. In addition to the usual diagnostic tools, there was a handheld computer for blood testing, and a portable chest x-ray machine.

Sitting in her own room in her favorite bedside chair, wearing her prettiest blue sweater, Katharine smiled at the doctor and seemed to enjoy the attention he was delivering. Experienced in the best ways to get along with Alzheimer's patients, this doctor moved slowly and spoke in calm, unhurried tones. Katharine responded by cooperating fully with the exam and blood work.

Sadly, the blood work revealed that Katharine's heart was failing. Additional blood testing identified that the cause of the heart failure was related to Katharine's failing kidneys, which had allowed impurities to build up in Katharine's blood. Her other organs were being slowly poisoned.

The doctor patiently explained our options. He said that without hospitalization, IV fluids, and kidney dialysis, Katharine would soon slide into a coma and shortly thereafter would die due to the cardiac instability that was already beginning. He said that the decision would be ours, whether we wanted her to be transported to the hospital for these procedures. He kindly added that our other option was to keep Katharine at home, making her comfortable until she died. He doubted that she would live more than a week.

My hesitation in making a decision about these options was a surprise even to me. Given that only two years before, I was calculating how many years might remain before Katharine would die, I was surprised to find that the choice was much more difficult than I would have thought. Dana arrived home from San Francisco on a late plane that Friday night, and we talked about our options. We knew that even with the hospitalization and treatment, we would only be prolonging the inevitable. The treatment held little hope for returning Katharine to a stable enough state to resume her life in our home and once again attend day care. We also knew that hospital treatment for Katharine would be traumatic. She was so happy in our home, and we knew that if we transported her again to the hospital, any sense of peace would again disappear.

Still, it was a difficult decision. As Catholics, we knew that the church neither condemns nor condones any particular technology used to care for those nearing death. Catholic teaching on end-of-life care is articulated in general principles on conserving human life, but the church does not specify particular treatment modalities that are mandated. For Catholics, a treatment is morally obligatory only when it holds out a reasonable hope of benefit for the patient, and is not excessively burdensome on that patient or on those responsible for the patient's care. While recent papal statements have made it clear that there is a general presumption in favor of providing nutrition and hydration to the patient, extraordinary measures were not morally obligated.

After a long discussion that evening, we decided to forego the extraordinary means we would need to maintain Katharine's life. We chose to keep Katharine at home and provide the comfort care we had already been providing. The doctor helped us to create a supportive environment for her. He ordered oxygen to be delivered to our home to aid Katharine's breathing, and diuretics to help reduce the fluid that was accumulating around her heart. We were confident that with his help, we could manage these last days of caregiving. The next morning, Katharine received the Sacrament of the Sick from our parish priest, and we all received Communion. It was a time of great sadness for us. The reluctant caregivers had surprisingly grown reluctant to give up the role.

Katharine remained awake all day Saturday. She petted Charli, who stayed with her all day, snuggling next to her on the bed. Throughout the day on Saturday, and into Sunday morning, Dana and I took turns feeding her all of her favorite foods, the chocolate pudding and ice cream she has always loved. However, by Sunday afternoon, she became unresponsive and died peacefully in her sleep at 8 A.M. Monday morning, just after Jonathan had left for school and Dana had left for work.

It was a strange feeling for me on that chilly Monday morning, to be sitting with Katharine in that newly quiet bedroom that I had become so familiar with during the previous three years. I had grown to know every corner of the room because of so many long and exasperating nights trying to convince Katharine to sleep. I realized how far we had come from those days of despair, to the days of hope and joy that Katharine finally brought to us. As I sat with her in the now lonely room on that dreary Monday, I realized that I was already missing her.

And, now, a year has passed since Katharine died. For a while I had trouble filling the extra hours. To care for Katharine, I had given up so much of my outside life. A teenager now, Jonathan is no longer wanting quite so much mothering. I still spend time with the women who helped us with Katharine in our home, and I volunteer to help other Alzheimer's families. Still, each afternoon at about 4 P.M., the time I used to pick up Katharine at day care, I catch myself looking at my watch, thinking that I must have to rush off from a meeting to drive to the center for Katharine. I am surprised to miss the ritual. I am surprised to miss her cheerful face each morning. I will always be grateful to Katharine for teaching us that no matter how "important" we may become in our jobs at work, it is always so much more important to care for those we love. While we learned that caregiving needs to be shared, we know now that caring for our parents, children, spouses, siblings, and friends is always going to be more important than our jobs. Caring for Katharine taught us that an evening spent by a sickbed will always last longer than the most brilliant theory on caregiving. We learned that even reluctant caregivers can learn to truly care.

Appendix: Resources

ORGANIZATIONS

The Alzheimer's Association

The mission of the Alzheimer's Association is to eliminate Alzheimer's disease through the advancement of research, while enhancing care and support services for individuals and their families. Their primary goal is to mobilize worldwide resources, set priorities, and fund select projects for biomedical, social, and behavioral research. A second goal is to promote, develop, and disseminate educational programs and training guidelines for health and social service professionals.

The Alzheimer's Association is invaluable to caregivers in facilitating access to services, information and optimal care techniques to maximize care and support for individuals and their families.

There are 200 chapters throughout the country. For information about your local chapter, contact the National Alzheimer's Association:

Alzheimer's Association
919 N. Michigan Avenue, Suite 1000
Chicago, IL 60611–1676
Web site: http://www.alz.org

The *Safe Return* Program

The Alzheimer's Association created the *Safe Return* Program to enable police and private citizens to identify people with Alzheimer's disease and help them return home quickly. *Safe Return* is a nationwide identification support and registration program that provides assistance to those who become lost locally or far away from home. When a person registered in *Safe Return* is lost, his or her family contacts the program's emergency number. Someone who finds a lost person can call the national number listed on the person's *Safe Return* identification bracelet (or necklace, clothing label or wallet card). Contact information for people registered in the program is stored in a national database, accessible 24-hours a day, 7 days a week.

For a *Safe Return* brochure and registration form, call: 800–272–3900

National Association of Area Agencies on Aging

A private nonprofit organization that provides information on the local Chapters of Area Agencies on Aging throughout the country. Contact them for information about transportation, legal aid, nutrition programs, housekeeping, senior center activities, counseling, and referral programs.

National Association of Area Agencies on Aging
1112–16th Street N.W.
Suite 100
Washington, DC 20036
202–296–8130

American Health Assistance Foundation

This Foundation is devoted to funding scientific research on Alzheimer's disease. However, the American Health Assistance Foundation's Alzheimer's Family Relief Program provides direct emergency financial assistance to Alzheimer's disease victims and caregivers when no other means are available. The Foundation also offers free educational materials on Alzheimer's disease upon request.

American Health Assistance Foundation
15825 Shady Grove Road
Suite 140
Rockville, MD 20850
301–948–3244

National Institute on Aging Information Center

A federal agency that provides free materials to the public, including fact sheets, pamphlets, and technical reports on Alzheimer's disease and other research on aging.

National Institute on Aging Information Center
P.O. Box 8057
Gaithersburg, MD 20898–8057
800–222–2225

SELECTED ALZHEIMER'S DISEASE-RELATED WEB SITES

In addition to the above resources, there are over 100 Web sites for Alzheimer's Caregivers. Sites that have been especially helpful to caregivers are included here.

Alzheimers.com

This is the best site I have found. It is a comprehensive online resource, updated daily, with the latest news and information about Alzheimer's disease and Alzheimer's care.

http://www.alzheimers.com

Alzheimer's Resource Center

The Mayo Clinic personnel offer information, explanations and advice about treatment and care for patients with Alzheimer's disease.

http://www/mayohealth.org/may/common/htm/alzheimers/htm

Alzheimers.com—Community Board and Support

Notes from hundreds of caregivers on techniques they have found useful for caring for loved ones with Alzheimer's disease.

http://www.alzheimers.com/cgi-bin/affinity

The Ribbon Online

A Web site inspired by *The Ribbon* newsletter, created to provide information for caregivers dealing with Alzheimer's. Back issues of *The*

Ribbon newsletter are available on this Web site. Chat rooms are available for caregivers and useful information sharing.

http://Theribbonwww.com

The Alzheimer's Association

The national Alzheimer's Association provides information about Alzheimer's disease, resources, research advances, publications and events. Includes links to local Alzheimer's Association chapters throughout the United States.

http://www.alz.org

A Year to Remember

This site provides Alzheimer's disease information and shares a personal story through poetry, photos, and a caregiver's journal. Message-board, links, resources.

http://www.zarcrom.com/users/yeartorem

Gerontology Institute

The Gerontology Institute provides seniors "Update on Aging" newsletter, video taped and live geriatric health care seminars on Alzheimer's disease, physical therapy, psychology and nutrition.

http://www/gerontologyinstitute.com

Alzheimer's Disease Education and Referral Center (ADEAR)

Information on Alzheimer's disease research, clinical trials, publications, bibliographic database, and links to other Federal resources. ADEAR is a service of the National Institution on Aging, National Institutes of Health.

http://www.alzheimers.org

TIME Slips

A site detailing stories told by patients with Alzheimer's disease. This is part of an artistic multi-city project.

http://www.timeslips.org/go.html

The Stages of Alzheimer's Disease

Information offered by the Institute for Brain Aging and Dementia.
http://www.alz.uci.edu/StagesAD.html

Alzheimer's Disease Resource Center

Medical news, information, links, message boards, books on Alzheimer's.
http://members.aol.com/healwell/alzheimers.htm

Bibliographic Essay

Until recently, families confronted with Alzheimer's disease had little access to information and support as there were few resources. While there were academic research reports on the origins and symptoms of the disease, there were few books that addressed the caregiving challenges that Alzheimer's patients present. Fortunately, the literature has begun to reflect the reality of the increase in Alzheimer's caregiving families. A growing number of new books have been published to assist the Alzheimer's family.

The following is an overview of selected books relating to Alzheimer's disease and caregiving. These books were chosen for inclusion because they were especially helpful either in providing information about successful care and management techniques, or in providing information from other caregivers who are experiencing similar challenges and emotions. The books are topically organized in an effort to assist the potential caregiver to find those books that will be of the most help in addressing their particular challenge. The first group of books include those which approach the subject of Alzheimer's disease from the professional point of view and provide information related to symptoms, treatment and behavioral strategies. The second group of books include those which explore the genetic foundations of the disease. While slightly more technical, caregivers can find valuable information about their family's risks of contracting the disease. The third group of books describe the ethical dilemmas that face the Alzheimer's caregiving family, and explore end-of-life dilemmas. The final and fastest growing group of books include memoirs written by family members of those suffering from Alzheimer's disease.

Each group of books provides support and information to the caregiving families. The books by professionals offer invaluable information and advice to potential caregivers, yet, few offer an acknowledgement of the emotional demands of caregiving. The memoirs offer a sympathetic voice and emotional support to the caregiver, yet, too often offer little practical help to the fledgling caregiver. For a full understanding of the disease, it is helpful to read books from each group.

ADVICE FROM THE PROFESSIONALS

The first group of books on Alzheimer's caregiving approach the subject from the point of view of urging readers to follow the professional's instructions in the diagnosis and treatment of Alzheimer's. In these books, there is excellent information yet little anecdotal information to help caregivers understand some of the emotions that they and other caregivers might be experiencing. The best example of one of these books is *The Thirty-Six Hour Day* (Baltimore, MD: Johns Hopkins Press, 1981,1991) by Nancy Mace and Peter Rabins. This book, which has sold over 500,000 copies, is widely regarded by those in the Alzheimer's caregiving community as the most comprehensive book to assist caregivers in learning about the disease and the demands of caregiving. Encyclopedic in its coverage of diagnosis and treatment, this book provides a reference for all caregivers. While invaluable, many caregivers have confided that *The Thirty-Six Hour Day* frightened them because of the graphic description of hallucinations, and behavior disorders that some Alzheimer's patients present. A second book that attempts to combine some of the strengths of *The Thirty-Six Hour Day* with practical suggestions for caregivers is *Alzheimer's Disease: A Guide for Families* (Reading, MA: Addison-Wesley Publishing Company, 1993). This book is valuable because it gives information about the emotional challenges faced by some caregivers. More recent books include, *Is It Alzheimer's?* (New York: Avon, 1998) by Roger Granet and Eileen Fallon which provides extensive, yet reassuring information about the symptoms of Alzheimer's that is especially helpful for the early stage, undiagnosed Alzheimer's patient. *Coping with Alzheimer's: The Complete Care Manual* by R. E. Markin (Secaucus, NJ: Citadel

Press, 1998) offers a unique perspective on the need to give attention to the legal, financial, medical and emotional needs of the Alzheimer's family. A former director of the Alzheimer's Research Foundation, Markin provides practical lists for the family of the Alzheimer's victim in this brief book. He stresses the need to address issues of power of attorney and financial needs early in the diagnosis process, and lists sources for health care equipment as well as information about arranging a funeral. Similarly, *When Someone You Love Has Alzheimer's* by Marilyn Larkin (New York: Dell, 1994) provides practical advice for the caregiving family. Larkin goes beyond Markin in providing a more comprehensive glossary and a listing of resources available to caregivers. Still, *Alzheimer's: The Complete Guide for Families and Loved Ones* by Howard Gruetzner (New York: Wiley, 1997) provides the most comprehensive information on treatment options. Gruetzner devotes an entire chapter to descriptions of psychiatric medications and dementia, and another chapter entitled "Treatment Possibilities."

To help the caregiver communicate with the patient, Harriet Hodgson offers *Alzheimer's: Finding the Words* (Minneapolis, MN: Cronimed, 1995). This book provides useful insights for communicating with one with a failing mind and offers valuable help on how to relate to an Alzheimer's patient when communication is a daily struggle. This guide shows how Alzheimer's affects speech, and gives proven, practical advice, based on life experience. Her book provides meaningful ways that caregivers can communicate even with a severely demented loved one by reminding readers that improving communication with a loved one is a way of showing respect for human dignity.

One of the most unique Alzheimer's caregiving books is one that is actually written for early stage Alzheimer's victims themselves. This book entitled *Alzheimer's: The Answers You Need* by Helen Davies and Michael Jensen (Forest Knolls, CA: Elder Books,1998) is the first guidebook directed to the actual victim of Alzheimer's disease and provides hopeful and encouraging reminders that an Alzheimer's sufferer can have a meaningful life after a diagnosis.

Finally, there is an excellent book directed to educating very young children about Alzheimer's disease. *Let's Talk About When Someone You Love Has Alzheimer's* by Elizabeth Weitzman (Center City, MN: Hazeldon, 1998) provides children with the same kinds of support offered to their parents.

RESEARCH ON GENETICS AND ALZHEIMER'S DISEASE

For the most up-to-date information on genetics and Alzheimer's, Joseph Rogers offers *Candle and Darkness* (Chicago, IL: Bonus Books, 1998). Dr. Rogers has devoted his entire scientific career to studies of aging and Alzheimer's disease and provides the reader with an accessible description of the current research on the correlates of Alzheimer's disease. This book is the first to offer comprehensive yet accessible coverage of Alzheimer's disease research for lay audiences. In addition to the valuable research information for families, Dr. Rogers cautions readers about the "dubious remedies" that many desperate families have attempted, and provides an extensive reading list for further information. In a related book, neurologist, Dr. Daniel Pollen provides readers with an understanding of the genetic causes of Alzheimer's in *Hannah's Heirs* (New York: Oxford University Press, 1996) by introducing readers to a family with a tragic multi-generational history of familial Alzheimer's disease. While *Hannah's Heirs* is written in a less accessible style than Rogers' book, it is engaging because it reads like a genetic detective story in determining who might be the next victim of the disease.

Does It Run In The Family: A Consumer's Guide to DNA Testing for Genetic Disorders by Doris Teichler Zallen (New Brunswick, NJ: Rutgers University Press, 1997) advises readers about the availability of genetic testing. Although not specifically targeted to Alzheimer's families, Dr. Zallen cautions readers to make informed decisions about testing for the susceptibility genes related to Alzheimer's disease.

ISSUES OF DEATH AND DYING

For a discussion on the ethics of treatment and end-of-life care for those with Alzheimer's disease, James and Hilde Lindemann-Nelson offer *Alzheimer's: Answers to Hard Questions for Families* (New York: Doubleday, 1996). Drawing from their research on moral issues of health care at the Hastings Center, this book presents hypothetical scenes that demonstrate some of the most common situations caregivers experience. This book is especially useful due to their exploration of end-of-life decision making. Related to this, Daniel Callahan, Director of the Hastings Center, offers *Setting Limits: Medical Goals in an Aging Society* (Washington, DC: Georgetown University Press, 1995). While not specifically targeted to those with Alzheimer's, this book provides invaluable information for caregivers navigating the health care system with their Alzheimer's impaired loved one. Similarly, Callahan's *The Troubled Dream of Life: In Search of a Peaceful Death* (New York: Touchstone, 1993) explores society's attempts to shape death. While he argues in favor of making choices regarding end-of-life treatment, Callahan argues persuasively against societal attempts to manage death through assisted suicide or euthanasia. M. Scott Peck presents a similar argument against euthanasia and assisted suicide in *Denial of the Soul* (New York: Harmony Books, 1997) as he explores the spiritual and medical perspectives on euthanasia and mortality. Although Peck does not specifically explore Alzheimer's disease, this book is helpful to the caregiver struggling with medical decisions at the final stages of the disease.

Sherwin Nuland's *How We Die* (New York: Vintage Books, 1993) presents a chapter on Alzheimer's disease. The chapter is illuminating because it not only describes the pathological changes associated with Alzheimer's disease, it also describes the devastation of the disease on the family. What is most valuable in Nuland's chapter is the explanation of why it is so difficult to understand the etiology of the disease. He acknowledges that the advancements in the biomedical aspects of the disease have not led to the discovery of any distinct cause of the disease, a method of curing it, or any way in which it may be prevented. Yet, Nuland's book is not without hope for such understanding.

From a different perspective, yet the same theme, *The Good Death* by Marilyn Webb (New York: Bantam Books, 1997) presents a brief case study of an Alzheimer's disease victim to illuminate current attempts to reshape the end of life. Death is presented as a peaceful respite from the ravages from the disease.

CAREGIVING MEMOIRS

The greatest value of the caregiving memoirs is to offer reassurance to caregivers that their experiences are shared by others. *Looking Ahead* by John Daniel (Washington, DC: Counterpoint Press, 1998) chronicles the caregiving journey of an adult son of an Alzheimer's victim. Written in a beautifully engaging style, Daniel documents his emotions as he provides devoted care to his demented mother and movingly describes the family conflict caused by the caregiving. Likewise, Julie Hildon's *The Bad Daughter* (Chapel Hill, NC: Algonquin Press, 1998) painfully describes the costs of caregiving as she narrates her decision to opt out of the caregiving role. She writes of the suffering that her mother's early onset disease caused during her teenage and early adult years. While the reader has a strong sense of the casualties of the disease, caregivers are given little hope to finding meaning in the caregiving. As is the case with *The Thirty-Six Hour Day, The Bad Daughter* may be depressing for the new caregiver.

Conversely, Ann Davidson's *Alzheimer's: A Love Story* (Secaucus, NJ: Birch Lane Press, 1997) offers a moving tribute to her Alzheimer's inflicted husband. In loving detail, she describes the difficulties they encounter, yet somehow manages to find meaning in the days they share. Likewise, Lela Knox Shank's book, *Your Name is Hughes Hannibal Shanks* (New York: Penguin Books, 1999) describes the fourteen year caregiving journey of the author. Shanks cared for her Alzheimer's impaired husband in their home until his death. This book is an especially helpful memoir because it not only describes the emotional journey, it also identifies the symptoms and stages of the disease and sets forth practical techniques for managing behavioral problems. Shanks clearly demonstrates that "the key to successful caregiving lies in never losing sight of the patient's humanity."

Less practical, yet no less moving is *The Painted Diaries* by Kim Zabbia (Minneapolis, MN: Fairview Press, 1996). This beautiful book offers a unique perspective on the disease through the use of art to explore the emotional struggles faced by the Alzheimer's patient and the patient's family. Color artwork throughout the book provides visual metaphors of the disease. Finally, a slightly more dated publication, reflecting out-dated information about the disease, yet a moving memoir is *Alzheimer's Disease: The Long Bereavement* by Elizabeth Forsythe (London: Faber and Faber, 1990).

Religious and spiritual themes emerge in *God Never Forgets* edited by Donald McKim (Louisville, KY: Westminster John Knox Press, 1997); *Alzheimer's: Making Sense of the Suffering* by Teresa Strecker (Layfayette, LA: Vital Issues, 1997); and in *A Time for Alzheimer's* by Florence Baurys (Houston, TX: Emerald Ink, 1998). For everyday spiritual reflections, *Coping with Caring* by Lyn Roche (Forest Knolls, CA: Elder Books, 1996) provides readers with inspiring daily readings. *Forgetting Whose We Are: Alzheimer's Disease and the Love of God* by David Keck (Nashville, TN: Abbington Press, 1996) provides the most theologically grounded perspective of Alzheimer's disease. In fact, Keck introduces Alzheimer's disease as the "theological disease" because the disease confronts us with a sustained dying. For Keck, Alzheimer's is an inescapable reminder that we will all die, and thus, the disease can be a mirror in which we can contemplate our own deaths.

Loss of control and death are always at the heart of Christian theological reflection, and Keck believes that Alzheimer's disease helps us to remember this.

The greatest strength of each of these books is to help readers find meaning in the disease through offering hope and spiritual guidance. While these inspirational books may not meet the needs of all caregivers, they can help those readers looking for spiritual guidance to make sense of the suffering from Alzheimer's.

The most recent, and surely most controversial memoir is *Elegy for Iris* by John Bayley (New York: St. Martin's Press, 1999). While this book recounts the life and Alzheimer's-related decline of his beloved spouse, philosopher, Iris Murdoch, the book has caused controversy for author, John Bayley. The controversy erupted over Bayley's willingness to reveal Murdoch's descent into dementia in this memoir. He describes the once-brilliant Murdoch's current fascination with what he sees as mindless activities. He describes her joy over children's television shows like the *Teletubbies*. Bayley also confesses his own frustrations and anger related to Murdoch's behavior. At one point in the book he recalls "giving her a surreptitious violent punch on the arm" when she acts inappropriately and creates a scene on a public bus. The response to the Bayley book by reviewers and readers has been mixed. While caregivers seem to appreciate Bayley's willingness to share the common emotions and frustrations of caregiving, there are critics who believe that Murdoch's dignity has been diminished through this portrayal of dementia. Still, for those who care for a loved one with Alzheimer's, Bayley's book is valuable because it movingly chronicles the loneliness of the caregiver who watches a much loved partner deteriorate.

Index

About the Author

ANNE HENDERSHOTT is Professor of Sociology at the University of San Diego. She has written and taught about work-family issues and is a frequent presenter at gerontology workshops and conferences.

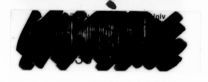

Date Due

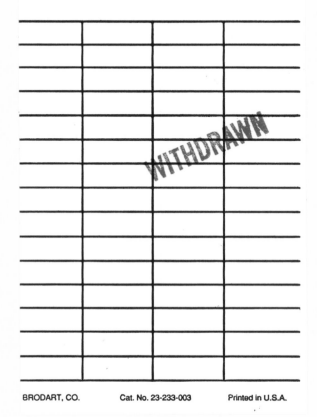